P9-DNC-400

THE CHEATER'S DIET

The Cheater's Diet

Lose Weight by
Taking Weekends Off

Paul Rivas, M.D.
with E. A. Tremblay

Health Communications, Inc.
Deerfield Beach, Florida

www.bcibooks.com

Library of Congress Cataloging-in-Publication Data
is available from the Library of Congress

©2005 Paul Rivas, M.D. and E. A. Tremblay
ISBN 0-7573-0321-8

Publisher: Health Communications, Inc.
          3201 S.W. 15th Street
          Deerfield Beach, FL 33442-8190

Cover design by Andrea Perrine Brower
Inside book design by Dawn Von Strolley Grove
Inside book formatting by Lawna Patterson Oldfield

Contents

Acknowledgments

I wish to acknowledge my entire office staff, especially Cricket, Joannie and Pat. Your loyal and tireless efforts over these many years are more appreciated than you'll ever know. You all are the reason our office works.

To my brother Mark Rivas—it's been the greatest pleasure working side by side with you. You make going to work even more fun than it already is.

Thanks to Ed Levien for his friendship, guidance and caring.

Thanks to another Ed—my terrific agent, Ed Claflin—for having faith in this book.

Ernie, you're the best medical writer for the layperson ever!

Tons of gratitude to Allison Janse, of Health Communications, Inc., for her discerning edits and wonderful guidance on this project.

A huge thank-you to Jeanette Tremblay for some truly inspired, not to mention delicious, recipes.

To my patients for believing.

Finally, to my three children, the most wonderful in the universe, Elizabeth, Sarah and David, and to my wife, Tammy. Without your love and support, everything would be meaningless and indeed would cease to exist.

Introduction

If you were told that from now on, you would have to work at a boring, repetitive job for sixteen hours a day, seven days a week, year after year, with a great starting salary, but no raises or bonuses, how long do you think you'd stick with it? Odds are you'd burn out within the first twelve months. Expecting to spend the rest of your life doing that kind of work is completely unrealistic. Yet this is exactly the kind of expectation we have of ourselves when we diet to lose weight.

Who can eat bland meals that contain no carbohydrates or fats for 365 days a year, every year for life? Who can live on a 1,500-calorie daily allotment with no relief in sight? No wonder 95 percent of dieters fail, with more than half of them quitting in the first six to twelve months. Diets are boring! Failure is built into them. And as you'll see in this book, even if you manage to stick with a diet over the long term, your body will eventually adjust to the changes you've made and start packing on weight again.

You avoid job burnout by adding variety to your work, taking time off and allowing yourself to have fun once in awhile. The good news is that you can do exactly the same thing with your diet. *You can take weekends off!* You can cheat with the foods you love most! And here's the bonus: Taking time off and allowing yourself to cheat on weekends helps you burn extra calories.

The Cheater's Diet not only encourages you, but *requires* you to cheat on weekends with delicious foods such as chocolate, wine, beer and pizza! That's right. During the workweek, you'll enjoy wonderful, satisfying meals that are designed to make you lose weight without giving up fat or carbohydrates. And on weekends, you get to choose any foods you like, from cake to steak. The Cheater's Diet allows you to say good-bye to deprivation and hello to guilt-free eating and cheating.

Best of all, it works.

How do I know? I've seen it. I'm a bariatrician—a physician who specializes in weight loss. In over a decade of practice, I've watched more than 15,000 patients struggle with their weight, try all kinds of diets and ultimately fail. I'm also a board-certified internist, so I'm concerned with more than getting my patients into smaller clothing sizes—their health is always my first concern. I don't believe that diets that cut carbs and allow you to eat all the saturated fat you want constitute a terribly good idea. Neither am I a big fan of food plans that cut your fat consumption almost to zero, but allow you to stuff yourself with white bread, rice and potatoes.

People who want to lose weight need a diet that puts the joy back into eating; doesn't require a lot of fuss, worry, guilt and sacrifice; beats the body's ability to adapt; offers lots of variety; and actually improves health. That's what the Cheater's Diet does. Of course, if you still insist on following the same old low-carb or low-fat plan that's been boring your palate for the past few months, the principles you read about here will work with them as well. Where weight management and health are concerned, there's a new golden rule: Cheaters *always* win, and winners *always* cheat. So read on, have fun, and *bon appétit*!

1

The Happy Ending That Could Be Yours

Once upon a time, Martha G., a woman in her mid-sixties from Baltimore, Maryland, was dangerously heavy. Like many people, she'd struggled with her weight for most of her life. She'd tried everything from addictive medications and calorie counting to food substitution programs and support groups. Nothing worked. She would lose the weight, then gain it right back. But Martha had heart. She wasn't ready to give up. She decided to have one more go at it.

This time she took a different approach. Instead of cutting carbs, fats or calories, she ate all the foods she loved: breads, pork roast, prime rib, mashed potatoes with gravy. Within a year, she shed forty-five pounds and showed no signs of gaining back her weight. It was my job to find out what was going on. Mind you, I'm not a detective. I'm a doctor.

What Goes Down Usually Comes Up

Nearly everything I know about losing weight I learned from my patients, and in my ten years of medical weight-loss practice, I have had over 15,000 teachers. They have taught me not to judge, but to encourage; not to preach, but to listen; not to push, but to guide. The first and most important lesson they offered, however, was simpler, more fundamental and very practical: Diets don't work!

Heresy, I know, but true nonetheless. Will a diet make you shed pounds? Of course. Almost any diet will make you thinner, whether you're cutting carbohydrates, reducing fat, controlling your portions or counting calories. Will it make you healthier? It may for the short term. But if in the long term it turns you into a weight-loss yo-yo—gaining and losing again and again—research has shown that you would have been healthier had you not lost weight in the first place. Therein lies the problem. All diets, by their very nature, turn you into a yo-yo.

Over 90 percent of all people who lose weight gain it back within two years. Study after study confirms it. The reason? Diets are boring. They take away your freedom of choice, and no matter how creative you are in the kitchen, giving up bread, steak and chocolate eventually makes you feel deprived. Then, when you cheat—and you will cheat—heaven help you. Is there any feeling worse than the guilt you get when you sneak a handful of cookies or devour a bowl of chocolate-chip ice cream?

After that happens, of course, you make a solemn promise to return to the rules of your diet. While the person across the table is devouring a Philly cheesesteak, you get to nibble on a turkey and cheese roll-up. When the person sitting next to you at the diner attacks a hot fudge sundae, you order a cup of coffee with a packet of sugar substitute. How many times does this have to happen before you throw in the towel and dive into the feast, only to come up for air six months later carrying all the pounds you had worked so long and hard to lose? Who can live that way, twenty-four hours a day, seven days a week, for an entire lifetime?

WHAT MAKES FAT DANGEROUS

It seems self-evident that carrying lots of extra weight puts more stress and strain on the body, and for a long time, many of us assumed that was the reason that overweight people tended to die younger of coronary disease. The heart had to work harder, so it wore out faster. Recent research, however, has told a very different story: Fat cells are little chemical factories that pump out all kinds of hormones. One of these, leptin, has become well-known for its role in controlling appetite. We're now aware of about twenty-five other hormones that fat cells generate, and more are discovered every year. The problem is, the more swollen with fat these cells get, the more hormones they pump out, and in this case, more is definitely not better. In large amounts, these chemicals constrict your blood vessels, allow fat to leak into your bloodstream, make your blood sugar and insulin levels rise, cause plaque to form on the inside of your arteries and even feed tumor cells. In fact, the American Cancer Society has estimated that obesity and being overweight lead to about 90,000 cancer deaths every year. In other words, fat is not simply a lump of inert yellow stuff that sticks like peanut butter to your insides. In excess, it is an active organ producing poisons that can kill you. Get rid of it. Maintain your weekday diet, and on weekends, cheat a little. If you do, you may gain an extra two to ten years of life.

To make matters worse, even if you manage to stay on a diet, sooner or later your body's metabolism will adjust by slowing down and saving more calories as fat, regardless of how little you eat. That's nature's way of keeping you safe from famine. If you want to keep off the weight, you'll eventually have to cut your intake to starvation levels. Ask anyone who has been on a carb-free diet for a couple of years about what happens when she adds even a single slice of bread to her daily fare. The pounds start piling back on, and they become more and more difficult to shed again.

So What Else Is New?

Such are the challenges my patients bring to my office. When I first opened my weight-loss clinic in 1994, I treated them in the same way that most doctors treat their overweight patients to this day: I told them to eat less. When they were unable to do that consistently, I gave them a stern lecture. Needless to say, my approach didn't work. After all, if you've fallen off a diet because it's boring, restrictive and ultimately ineffective, what is the point of a doctor telling you to get back on it?

My patients required a new approach. Some asked for medications, and I began to prescribe them. Medicine has come a long way since the days of fen-phen and addictive amphetamines. For many people, the modern appetite suppressants I prescribe offer a dependable and effective way to maintain a healthful weight. But pills aren't for everyone. They're expensive, they're not covered by most insurance plans, and the idea of staying on them for life makes many people uncomfortable.

So I scoured the literature, looking for some fresh approach to help people control their weight. Believe me, there is not a new diet, weight-loss organization or peer-reviewed study that I haven't closely investigated. Guess what I found: The new diets are variations of the old diets. The organizations, while providing great support to their members, don't offer innovative ideas for weight loss and maintenance, and most studies lead to tantalizing theories about what new therapies might be available years from now.

Because my patients were not willing to wait for science to provide an answer that might or might not appear in the hazy future, they took matters into their own hands.

A Lesson Learned

The fact is, many of them had already found the answer I was looking for. Martha was a good example. When she came to me, her blood studies were normal—she hadn't developed any of the many health problems that often plague overweight people, such as diabetes and high cholesterol—but she had a strong sense of pride in herself and her appearance. Carrying extra pounds made her feel as if she were "letting herself go."

She was strongly motivated to lose weight.

I made my usual recommendations, which included eating meals that were low in fat and had low to moderate amounts of carbohydrates. When she came for a return visit, I asked how her eating habits were shaping up. She looked a little sheepish.

"I cheated. I had a couple of drinks on the weekend," she told me.

A glass or two of wine, I wondered, or maybe a bottle of beer?

"No," she said, "vodka tonics. I've heard they're lowest in calories."

This is a moment that eventually comes to nearly everyone who tries to lose weight: the admission that they've been eating or drinking something they shouldn't. In other words, they've been cheating.

My response to Martha was the same one I give to all my patients. I told her it was okay to fall off the wagon now and then, that having a drink, a slice of cake or a scoop of ice cream on a weekend wouldn't affect her weight, so long as she got right back up and returned to her food plan. I knew from experience that people who deprive themselves of their favorite foods in order to follow a weight-loss diet are the mostly likely to give up.

So part of my job, as I see it, is to encourage them, again and again, to go easy on themselves. Eating a cupcake is not a sin, no matter how guilty you feel for doing it or how guilty those around you try to make you feel. Sometimes, polishing off that ice-cream cone is an idea whose time has come.

Eventually, that encouragement began to pay off in ways I hadn't expected. A pattern was emerging among my patients.

After being reassured that breaking the rules now and then wasn't such a terrible thing, some of them started to cheat on a regular basis. They allowed themselves one or two days a week when they relaxed the rules and pretty much ate anything they liked. They didn't binge, but they indulged in second helpings at meals or ate foods from the "forbidden" list—the fatty ones, the starchy ones, the sweet ones.

What surprised me was that not only did these patients experience no reversals or plateaus in their weight loss, but they actually lost weight *faster* than patients who didn't cheat on a regular basis. And they were far more likely to stick with their food plans over long periods of time.

It was time to do more research, this time not on dieting but on cheating. As it turned out, others around the country were seeing similar results. Dr. Tedd Mitchell, medical director of the Cooper Wellness Center in Dallas, was having great success using his 80/20 rule. That is, he was instructing his patients to eat healthful, wholesome, low-fat meals 80 percent of the time and to eat whatever they liked 20 percent of the time. That translates into four days on and one day off. Barbara Crosby, a nutrition researcher in Valley Stream, New York, had women add an extra 500 calories a day to their meals on weekends and claims they were burning up to 10,000 extra calories per week.

"I eat lots of chicken, fish, salads and vegetables during the week," Martha said. "And I eat some bread, usually wholewheat. During the week, it's not hard to be good. But I really enjoy eating, and I look forward to the weekends when I can let myself cheat now and then."

Martha's doing exactly what she should be doing. She's

treating her weight loss and maintenance like a job. Five days a week, she's very strict with herself. She eats wholesome, tasty food, but she watches her portion sizes and is careful not to overdo fats and carbs. On weekends, she takes time off and has fun. She comes from a German family and loves traditional ethnic dishes, so on weekends chicken is not always her first choice from the menu. She treats herself to wonderful breads and mashed potatoes, and, of course, still has the occasional vodka and tonic. Martha also has a sweet tooth. "I love anything made with white flour or sugar," she said. Most importantly, Martha loves the way she looks and feels now. "You'd never know I was sixty-eight," she said. She loves the way she eats, too.

I must mention that Martha doesn't exercise. She has rheumatoid arthritis, which restricts the kinds of movements she can do. Exercise should be an integral part of everyone's life. There is no doubt that it makes you healthier and stronger, helps prevent many diseases and, of course, makes you look better. But as we'll see, what it doesn't do is make you lose weight—unless you put in at least one hour of vigorous movement every day. Few people have the time or energy to do that. However, there is a way to use physical activity to help you lose weight, which we'll discuss later.

So let's admit it: Food is fun! Not only do we enjoy eating, but we take great joy and pleasure in the camaraderie of feasting at a table with family and friends. If we spend every single day of our lives trying to be Spartans and denying ourselves these pleasures, why have a life at all? The good news is, like Martha, you can enjoy your pleasure foods and still achieve healthful results. Let's find out how.

2

Overcoming Obesity: If You're Fat, It's Not Your Fault

We're not supposed to be fat. That's not what nature wants for us. But we're not supposed to be down-to-the-bone skinny, either. Your fat layer should be more like a thin, comfortably fitting life jacket than a blown-up inner tube, and in a way, it has the same use—to preserve your life.

Fat stores energy, and energy comes from food. That energy is what we call "calories." Undoubtedly, you're all-too-familiar with the word, but you needn't make a cross with your fingers as if you were fending off a vampire every time you hear it. Without calories, you couldn't survive.

When you eat, your body takes carbohydrates and fats, which are chock-full of calories, out of your food and floats them down your bloodstream. The carbohydrates are in a form of sugar called glucose. As your blood becomes sweeter and sweeter, the sugar-removal system in your body switches on, and your pancreas begins to manufacture a hormone called insulin. Insulin carries the calorie-rich sugar out of your system and puts it in three places: your liver and your muscles (in a form called glycogen), and your fat cells, where the saturated-food fats you consume are also stored. As the fat cells begin to expand like little balloons, lo and behold, your belly, butt and thighs begin to grow. Why does your body do this to you? Because calories are like gasoline to your internal motor—it can't run without them.

Your body, understandably, is concerned about that. Remember, there was a time when grocery stores didn't exist, and people had to run around the woods with bows and arrows, hoping to bag a meal before it skittered to safety up a tree. Eating was literally a hit-or-miss affair. Sometimes it happened, and sometimes it didn't. And sometimes it didn't for a long time.

As it turned out, our bodies were pretty smart and developed a way to store fat as fuel during times of abundance so you could use it when pickings were a little leaner. How ingenious! Fat was portable, efficient and dependable. And as an added benefit, it could help keep you warm in cold weather.

WHAT IS LEPTIN?

If you've read much about weight loss, you've probably bumped into the word "leptin." Leptin is a hormone that's secreted by fat cells and then travels by way of the bloodstream to the brain. There it acts as a signal that the body has stored enough energy as fat, and it's time to burn some. The brain then tells the body, "Okay, go for it."

Leptin was first discovered about ten years ago by researchers at Rockefeller University. A couple of years later, researchers at the University of Georgia showed that leptin's signal didn't just cause a reduction in the size of fat cells; it actually caused them to die—which explained why lab rats remained thin long after the experiment had stopped. Recent studies show that leptin ultimately transforms normal fat cells into little fat-burning furnaces before they give up the ghost. With the discovery of leptin, hope was high in the beginning that we had at last found the key to controlling weight loss. However, human metabolism has proven a bit more complicated than rat metabolism, so a working medication based on the hormone has yet to be developed.

That was then, but this is now. Human physiology hasn't quite caught on to the fact that lunch no longer depends on accurate aim or a great crop of nuts and berries during the foraging season. In fact, with modern methods of food production and distribution, few of us in the United States ever miss the midday meal—or the other two, for that matter. And, of course, there are all those snacks in between.

So we eat and eat, and we keep storing more and more fat, because those lean times, when we would naturally use up our stores, never come. That's really bad for us. It increases our risk of heart attack, stroke, high blood pressure, diabetes, arthritis and several types of cancer. In our culture, it can also make us less attractive to other people, which can have terrible consequences for self-esteem. Why, then, do we eat so much?

With a Flip of the Hunger Switch

We eat because we're hungry. Surprised? Somehow, I didn't think you would be. But to say we eat from hunger isn't really an answer that tells us much. For that, we have to dig a little deeper. We have to explain why we are hungry and what exactly hunger is.

You may think that being hungry is the feeling your stomach gives you when it's empty. Good guess, but not exactly true. It's more accurate to say that hunger is the signal your brain gives you that it's time to eat. How does your brain know? It gets lots of complex signals from the body and the bloodstream, which cause temporary chemical imbalances in the part of the brain that controls your appetite. That flips on what I call the "hunger switch." The brain wants to get back into balance. The body wants to get back into balance. The blood wants to get back into balance. All that balance depends on food. So you eat something, and all is right with the world. The muscles get all the energy they need; you consume exactly the amount you need in order to sate yourself; and your hunger goes away. Except that sometimes it doesn't.

When All Is Not Right with the World

Sometimes, even a stomach stretched tight by a five-course meal doesn't signal that feeling of satisfaction that tells you you've had enough. You feel so uncomfortable that you'd like to unbutton your pants, yet you still want to eat. What's going on?

Something in the thermostat is out of whack. When everything is supposed to be in balance, it isn't. You have too little of those chemicals (neurotransmitters) in your brain, and until you manufacture enough to flip off the hunger switch, you're going to continue feeling hungry. And as long as you feel hungry, there's a very good chance you'll keep eating.

Now, the problem with hunger is not just that it makes you eat more. It also makes you get fatter faster. When you're ravenous, your system understands the feeling as a signal that there's a problem afoot. From your body's point of view, the situation seems something like this: *She's eating, but I'm not feeling it. She must not be eating enough. If she's not eating enough, maybe there isn't much food around. Just to be on the safe side, I'd better be careful about the way I'm spending calories. In fact, I'd better put away as many as I can for even leaner days that may be coming.*

In order to do that, you become very efficient in the way you use fuel, as if you have suddenly transformed from being a gas-guzzling SUV into a subcompact that gets fifty miles per gallon. You do this in a couple of ways. First, you slow down your basal metabolism, which is the rate at which you use energy for normal, internal processes when you're not doing anything but sitting on the couch and watching yet another boring reality TV show. Then you start socking away energy in your fat cells instead of delivering it to your muscles for immediate use. This, unfortunately, encourages an expanding waistline and discourages the formation of beautiful, lean muscle. The net result: The hungrier you are when you eat, the more likely you are to gain weight from the meal.

The Willpower Paradox

You can see the problem. If you go on a calorie-sparing diet, you make yourself hungrier and hungrier. The more that happens, the better your body gets at storing energy as fat. Of course, it has to give up some of its stores eventually, just to keep you going day to day. That's why you're able to lose weight—although probably more slowly than you'd like. But something else happens that's a little more sinister: When you shed pounds, they don't all represent fat. Some of those pounds—as many as half—come from muscle. That's right. Your body begins to cannibalize itself. It considers fat stores so important to survival that it actually uses up muscle fiber to feed its energy needs.

Muscle, of course, is important. For one thing, the less of it you have, the slower your basal metabolism becomes and the more energy you store instead of burn. But beyond that, less muscle means more sugar-bearing insulin gets turned away—

and guess where most of the sugar it carries ends up? In your fat tissue.

The effect of all this is that once you lose weight and begin to gain it back, you're more likely to replace lost muscle with fat. Your slower metabolism makes it more difficult to lose weight again. The process takes longer, and you probably won't be able to lose as much. And every time you yo-yo, the situation gets worse.

Okay, then, you say to yourself, once you take off some weight, you just won't let yourself gain it back. You'll discipline yourself to stay on your diet for the rest of your life, and that will be that. There's one problem. "That" won't be that.

Your Body's Set Point

Over 90 percent of all people who lose weight on a diet gain it back, plus a little extra, within two years. Now, while it may be true that nine out of ten people simply don't have the self-restraint to continue restricting their food intake indefinitely (and if that's true, you can't blame them . . . who wants to look forward to a lifetime of restrictive eating?), the fact is, no matter how self-controlled we are, many of us have genes that won't allow us to lose a large amount of weight and keep it off. Everyone has a predisposition to maintain a certain weight, and unless you restrict food consumption to starvation levels, the body eventually becomes so extremely efficient at putting away calories that you begin to gain back pounds even if you don't eat more. And let's face it: At some point, you're going to start eating more because your body isn't going to take the abuse of your dieting. It will fight back. It will make you hungrier and hungrier. So while it gets better and better at increasing your girth with the little bit of food you allow, it also gets more and more insistent in its demand for more consumption. A double whammy!

WHO IS OBESE?

When we think about the word "obese," it can conjure pictures of people who weigh so much that they have trouble standing up. Medically, however, you can be considered obese at much lower weights. One effective way to determine whether you are obese or not is to calculate your body mass index (BMI). Multiply your weight in pounds by 705. Divide that by your height in inches, then divide it by your height in inches again. If the number falls between 25 and 27, you're overweight. From 27 to 30, you're obese. Over 30, you're seriously obese. However, if you're extremely muscular or over 70 years old, these numbers may not apply to you, and they don't if you're younger than 18. A quicker way to test for obesity may simply be to measure your waistline. Men who measure 40" and women who measure 35" around the midsection are considered obese and at serious risk for heart disease.

It's important to note that you really do just gain the weight back, with maybe a little extra. Most people won't keep gaining indefinitely. People reach a set point, which is a phrase used to signify the weight at which your body feels comfortable and safe from starvation. It's the weight to which your internal thermostat is set, and once you reach it, your hunger switch flips off. The problem faced by overweight and obese people is that their set point is too high.

Thanks for the Fat Genes, Mom and Dad

Many overweight and obese people are genetically predisposed to having a high set point. This means two things. First, you inherited a tendency toward being overweight, though you can only fulfill that tendency under the right conditions. For example, you must live in a place where food is readily available. Second, you're particularly vulnerable to certain triggers—things or events that cause your internal thermostat to reset—in your environment, including stress, medications, sugar binges, illness, alcohol, poor nutrition, hormonal fluctuations and many more.

You can see the dramatic effects of these triggers and conditions among people who come to the United States from cultures where obesity is rare. Before you know it, these folks find themselves moving into plus-size wardrobes. The condition and trigger, in this case, are probably one and the same: exposure to an overabundance of food, especially junk food.

You can see something similar developing in other countries that have imported some elements of our lifestyle. Fast food is now readily available in Brazil, for example, and obesity is rapidly turning into a national health problem there—this in a country where maintaining a beautiful, thin body has traditionally been a national fetish. A recent survey showed that 40 percent of Brazilian adults are overweight, and one in ten is obese. The average set point has gone up, and once a set point goes up, it rarely comes down.

Are You an Emotional Eater?

Many people believe they eat because of emotional stress, that food relieves depression or fills an emotional void inside of them. Some even talk about "stuffing" their feelings.

I'm not here to tell them that they're wrong, because in a way, they're not. They're accurate when they say that their binges coincide with bad moods, arguments with significant others, traumatic events or crushing disappointments. And I won't disagree that sometimes consuming a half-gallon of ice cream seems to calm inner turmoil. But why do we choose to eat rather than perform some other activity in reaction to emotional stress? Why not build a model airplane, wash the car or rob a bank?

Here's an interesting fact: A low serotonin level in the brain can make you feel depressed. It can also make you feel hungry. Eating certain foods, like sugar and starch, helps restore serotonin to a higher level. Bringing the brain's chemistry back into balance in this manner also relieves depression. So *voilà*, we know why some people "stuff" their feelings.

You can get that same effect, by the way, through vigorous physical activity. Several studies have confirmed that exercise is as powerful as medication in relieving mild-to-moderate depression, so if you're feeling down, a brisk walk may help you as much as a gallon of chocolate-chip ice cream.

If you feel that you often overeat during moments of crisis, stress or depression, you're probably right, and eating is certainly one way—although not a particularly healthful one—to ease those nasty feelings. However, as you've just learned, you don't eat because you're depressed. You eat because you're hungry.

Outsmarting Your Body

The body wants what it wants, and what it wants is to maintain its weight at its set point. As noted, the set point keeps you from starving during times when food is hard to come by. When you try to defeat the set point, your body does everything in its power to convince you of the folly of your ways, and if you remain unconvinced, it will snatch the wheel out of your hands and take over the driving. Evolution is powerful. It exerts its will through inherited genes, and woe unto you if you try to resist it through willpower.

That's why I mean it when I say that if you're fat, it's not your fault. In fact, if you're like most overweight people, you have probably shown more willpower than any thin person ever has or ever will. Don't believe it? Add up all the pounds you've lost throughout your life, even if you've gained them back again. You've probably lost, in total, several times your current weight, and you did it all through self-discipline and self-denial. That took courage and fortitude. Unfortunately, nobody told you that every time you came close to the goal line, the rules of the game would force you to back up again. So what should you do?

I said before that the human body is smart and wants what it wants. Now I'm going to tell you something that's even more important: You're smarter than your body. You can get it to behave in exactly the way that you want it to. You can make it get thin and like being that way. But you can't do it with willpower. That's like trying to win a tug-of-war with an elephant by using your brute strength. It just isn't going to happen. If, however, you use your intelligence and come up with an idea like tying your end of the rope to a bulldozer, you have a shot. That's using your head. Like your body, elephants are smart. They can even do tricks! However, they're not in the same league as you. So the key is to figure out how to use your native intelligence to defeat the strengths of your body's genetic code.

Fooling Your Genes

Your body has two powerful weapons at its disposal: the ability to make you feel famished and the ability to make you feel bored.

On most weight-loss diets, boredom kicks in first. Why? Because they're either based on completely restricting you from certain foods, or they're so Draconian in the way you have to control your portions that you finally throw up your hands and dive into the pasta carbonara. (For the uninitiated, that's spaghetti made with cream and bacon or ham. And it is, to put it bluntly, to die for.)

Who wants to live that way? Variety is the spice of life! We're made to enjoy diversity in what we eat, and when we don't get it, we move on. The average dieter in the United States remains on a diet for six weeks. Need I say more?

Perhaps, though, you're not average. Maybe, unlike most people, you have a high tolerance for boredom, and you feel so extremely motivated by health and cosmetic concerns that you can ignore the tedium and forge ahead. What's the big payoff for all of this indomitable willpower? Your metabolism starts housing nearly every calorie you consume in a fat cell. Or you can take an approach that's a hundred times more fun and effective. You can cheat. In fact, if you do it right, cheating can actually make you lose weight faster.

That probably contradicts everything you've ever been told about losing weight. In fact, you've probably been made to feel that you should hang your head in shame every time you sneak something into your mouth that your diet strictly forbids. Well, don't.

The idea is simple. Think about it in terms of taking a vacation or of just taking weekends off from a job. If you forced yourself to slave every waking hour of every day of the week, you would burn out pretty quickly. You wouldn't be much good for your own purposes or anyone else's. Your efficiency would drop, your alertness would fall, and your energy would plummet. On the other hand, taking Saturday and Sunday off to relax and gather your resources actually makes you *better* at your job when you return on Monday. You're rested and ready to go, with all pistons pumping.

Losing weight is no different. If you take a couple of days off every week, you'll find that when you return to your diet, you'll burn off pounds at an amazing rate. As we've seen, when you lessen the amount of food you eat, your body soon adjusts by slowing down basal metabolism and storing calories rather than burning them. You'll still lose weight for a while, but very slowly. Eventually, you'll plateau, and unless you become an absolute tyrant about your caloric intake, that's where you'll stay—until the body becomes so efficient at storing calories that you start putting pounds back on again.

This scenario may sound like bad news, but, in fact, it contains the solution to the twin problems of slow metabolism and boredom. Here's the clue: Although the body adjusts, it can't do so instantly. It takes a day or two. You can stay ahead of the body's natural behavior by changing your eating pattern every so often. If, during the week, you consume a diet that requires portion control and contains a low-to-moderate amount of fat and carbohydrates, the body will gradually turn down the heat in its fat burner. If, however, you then suddenly raise your caloric intake for a couple of days—say, over the weekend—alarm bells go off and your metabolism turns the heat back up. It thinks it doesn't need to store so many calories and begins to burn them up at a much faster rate. When you change directions yet again at the end of the weekend and suddenly cut your intake back while your metabolism is still burning fuel like a rocket, your body will have to find its fuel supply in some place other than the food you just ate, and that place would be . . . yes, your body fat.

3

Weekend Pleasures

L et's get to the good part first. Let's say you've just come off a week on some diet or other—low-carb or low-fat or low-calorie—and it's Saturday morning. The weekend at last! In an ideal world, you would have two days to sleep late, lounge around the house, go out to dinner, maybe even see a movie. In the real world, unfortunately, the house needs cleaning, you have to cheer your kids through their soccer games, your in-laws are coming for Sunday dinner, and the front lawn is waiting for the mower.

Cheer up. There's good news. Eating is going to be fun! Over the next two days, you'll free yourself from restrictions, food groups and healthful choices, and develop such a fondness for your fridge that it will seem like the best ride in Disney World.

Your Weekend Cheat Sheet: The Rules of Healthful Cheating

No matter which diet you're following, you *must* cheat for two consecutive days out of every week. Actually, you should limit your cheating time to about thirty-six hours, which comes to a day and a half. Start cheating at 9 A.M. on Saturday; stop at 9 P.M. on Sunday. During that time, you need to add calories to your diet to stoke your metabolism. There are two easy ways of going about this.

First, you can simply eat a lot more of what you have been eating during the week. If you feel like calculating calories, figure that each day you'll need to consume an extra ten calories for every pound you weigh. If you weigh a hundred pounds, add 1,000 calories to your diet. If you don't want to do the math, either use the table below as a guide or just take second helpings.

Weight in lbs.	Extra Calories Needed
100	1,000
120	1,200
140	1,400
160	1,600

Weight in lbs.	Extra Calories Needed
180	1,800
200	2,000
220	2,200
240	2,400

The second way is to add new items to your menu—in fact, add anything you like. Unless you have a health problem, such as diabetes or heart disease, that restricts which types of foods you can eat (always follow your doctor's advice), the only rule is this: Do not eat "binge" foods. If you can't stop eating ice cream until the entire gallon is gone, skip the ice cream. Got to inhale that entire bag of potato chips rather than just munch a handful? Sorry. Potato chips aren't for you.

Otherwise, indulge yourself with the most sinful, forbidden foods you like. I'm talking pizza, ice cream, peanut butter, chocolate, wine and all the other "health" foods you crave all week long. That's right, I said health foods. When people try to make you feel guilty for eating or drinking that comfort food on the weekend, here's what you tell them.

Pizza

Not only does pizza taste great, but it may also be the closest thing we have to a miracle food. Its sauce contains the highest concentration of lycopene, a powerful antioxidant, of any food that reaches Americans' plates, and the fat in the cheese is what delivers the lycopene efficiently to your system. Here are some ways you can benefit from lycopene:

- **Cut your risk for heart attack and stroke.** The ongoing Women's Health Study at Harvard University, which has been following the health of 40,000 women for the past eleven years, reports that women who ate seven or more meals containing tomato dishes (including pizza) each week lowered their risk for cardiovascular disease by 30 percent.
- **Prevent tumors of the digestive tract.** Researchers in Milan, Italy, claim that regular consumption of pizza can lower your risk for cancer of the mouth by 33 percent, cancer of the esophagus by almost 60 percent, and colon cancer by 25 percent. In a review of seventy-nine studies of lycopene, the *Journal of the National Cancer Institute* stated that research showed a strong link between consuming lycopene and lowered risk for cancer of the stomach, pancreas and rectum.
- **Protect the prostate.** Good news for men! A now-famous Harvard Medical School study found that men who ate ten or more servings a week of tomato sauce (on pizza or pasta) or strawberries, which also contain lycopene, lowered their risk of developing prostate cancer by 45 percent. Men who ate four to seven servings lowered their risk by 20 percent.
- **Protect the female reproductive system.** Good news for women! A study published in the *International Journal of Cancer* reported that lycopene, in the form of two half-cup servings of tomato sauce a week, significantly reduced the risk for ovarian cancer in pre-menopausal women. (The same study showed that eating five carrots a week reduced the risk for ovarian cancer in post-menopausal

women.) A study at Harvard pinpointed the risk reduction at 40 percent. The *Journal of the National Cancer Institute* reported that lycopene also has benefits in preventing breast and cervical cancer.

• **Keep you breathing.** Good news for smokers and ex-smokers! The review in the *Journal of the National Cancer Institute* also reported a strong association between high levels of lycopene in the bloodstream and lowered risk for lung cancer. If you want to reduce your risk to its lowest level, though, don't smoke.

Obviously, you shouldn't eat pizza every day. It's full of fat, salt and calories, which would quickly start to pile on the pounds. But as a weekend treat, it's one of the best you can give yourself. To boost the positive health effects even more, make your own pizza shells with whole-grain flour (or cook whole-grain pasta), which will add fiber to your meal.

By the way, what's been said about pizza is also true of pasta with red sauce, although the concentration of lycopene in pizza sauce tends to be higher. If you follow the Cheater's Diet's weekday plan (chapter 4), you can have small portions of white pasta during the week, and even make an entire meal of it on Saturday or Sunday.

Wine

Mankind has been fermenting grapes to create wine for more than eight thousand years. Wines have found their way into cuisines, religions, romance and mythology. People collect wines, trade them and celebrate with them. Who hasn't raised a glass on occasion to toast the health of a friend? Well, it's no wonder. Louis Pasteur once said, "Wine can be considered . . . the most healthful and most hygienic of all beverages." Study after study shows that he was right. Wine, especially red varieties such as pinot noir and cabernet, contains high levels of antioxidants called polyphenols as well as an estrogen-like substance called resveratrol. Resveratrol can provide you with antioxidant, anticoagulant, anti-inflammatory and anti-cancer effects. Here's what red wine can do for you:

- **Raise your level of good cholesterol.** Researchers in France found that consumption of red wine not only increases HDL (high-density lipoprotein) cholesterol, the type that actually removes dangerous plaque from your arteries, but also creates a type of HDL that contains particles rich in components that play a protective role in heart disease.

- **Keep your heart soft and supple.** Conditions such as high blood pressure and heart failure can cause the heart to become hard and stiff, so that it has a more difficult time pumping blood. Resveratrol, the substance found abundantly in red wine, helps fight this effect. It also helps prevent blood clotting in the arteries, a condition that causes heart attacks and can lead to sudden death.

- **Protect against certain cancers.** Doctors at the University of Santiago de Compostela in Spain have conducted research that suggested wine may have some protective effect against lung cancer. Researchers at the University of Virginia have come to similar conclusions, and many studies have shown that the resveratrol in wine may help prevent other kinds of cancer.

- **Keep your brain healthy.** In 2002, *Neurology,* the scientific journal of the *American Academy of Neurology,* published a study that showed red-wine drinkers were half as likely as non-drinkers to develop various kinds of dementia, including Alzheimer's disease. Other studies suggested that red wine (and fresh grapes) may have a protective effect against strokes.

DR. FRANK'S PINOT NOIR

All red wines contain antioxidants called polyphenols, as well as resveratrol, a substance that grapes and some other plants manufacture to fight off fungi. White wines don't contain it because the skin of the grapes used to make them, which contains all the health-promoting chemicals, is removed before the fruit is fermented. Not all red wines are created equal, however. Many tests have shown that pinot noir wines have the highest concentrations of resveratrol, and of the pinot noirs, one stands out head and shoulders above every other wine in the world: Dr. Konstantine Frank's Fleur de Pinot Noir, from vineyards in the Finger Lakes region of New York. According to Professor Leroy L. Creasy, who conducted an eight-year study of New York wines for Cornell University, pinot noir grapes contain a lot of resveratrol because they have thin skins and grow in tight clusters, making them a likely target for fungi. Dr. Frank's wine, however, contains an unusual amount of the substance, even for pinot noir. One bottle contains the equivalent of 17,000 resveratrol supplement capsules (over $8,000 worth)! If you can't find Fleur de Pinot Noir, which costs about $18 a bottle, Winery Lake Pinot Noir, from Sterling Vineyards, is a good choice for around $20, and Echelon Pinot Noir is a great buy for around $13.

Of course, don't drink wine if you have a problem with drinking alcohol to excess. Moderate drinking generally means no more than two five-ounce glasses of wine a day for men and no more than one for women.

Chocolate

The day of the chocoholic is here! In moderate amounts, chocolate is one of the most healthful gifts you can give to yourself. It's extremely high in flavonols (a type of antioxidant), and it's chock-full of vitamins and minerals. In fact, it's so good for you that people who eat chocolate three times a month live, on average, a year longer than people who don't.

There is one caveat, however. You get the most benefit from eating the highest-quality chocolate, which means it has a high cocoa content—at least 70 percent. That leaves out milk chocolate and white chocolate (which, to purists, isn't *real* chocolate). As a rule, the darker the better. Look for cocoa content on the label. If it's not there, find another brand. Specifically, chocolate:

- **Supplies you with magnesium.** Cocoa is the richest known natural source of magnesium. Among its many other roles in the human body, magnesium keeps your muscles and nerves functioning normally, helps maintain the rhythm of your heartbeat, supports your immune system, aids in making your bones strong, helps regulate your blood-sugar levels and aids in keeping your blood pressure low.
- **Helps thin your blood.** One study showed that drinking twenty-five grams (one ounce) of cocoa can prevent blood platelets, in the same way small doses of aspirin do, from sticking together or forming dangerous clots.

DOVE® DARK CHOCOLATE

While the cocoa content is important in choosing a chocolate, so is the way the cocoa has been processed. Processing can destroy many of the antioxidants that are present in raw cocoa beans. The most healthful, easily obtainable and delectable chocolate I've found is Dove Dark, made by Mars. Mars has developed a proprietary processing method, called Cocoapro, which almost completely retains the super-high levels of antioxidants that are naturally present in chocolate.

Dove Dark is so rich in antioxidants that it's actually been used in medical research. Just eat it or make a great hot chocolate with it. Heat up a cup of milk in your microwave, then place two pieces of Dove Dark into the milk, let them melt, then stir. If you can't find Dove Dark, try Valrhona Guanaja, a French chocolate available at most Trader Joe's stores; or Starbucks Dark Deliciously Chunky Chocolate, available at Starbucks Coffee. True chocolate lovers are aware of all the other wonderful choices out there, which include handmade chocolates from around the world.

Cocoa doesn't have the same harsh side effects as aspirin, such as gastrointestinal bleeding, but the beneficial effects don't last as long.

- **Destroys free radicals.** Free radicals are oxygen molecules in the bloodstream that can cause oxidation damage to cells in the same way they can cause rust on metal. When they combine with cholesterol molecules, they cause the cholesterol to form plaque on the inside of arteries, which can lead to a heart attack or stroke. They can also damage cells in a way that causes cancer. Antioxidants swallow those oxygen molecules and render them harmless. Cocoa offers some of the highest known concentrations of antioxidants of any food, more than three times the concentration present in green tea, according to researchers at Cornell University.

• **Controls your blood pressure.** One study discovered that people who drink cocoa show more nitrous-oxide activity in their blood. Nitrous oxide is critical to controlling blood pressure.

As with many cheat foods, chocolate does have its downside if you eat too much of it, especially in the form of chocolate bars. Eating more than two ounces a day may get you into the danger zone where fat and sugar are concerned. And even pure cocoa powder, which has far less fat and no added sugar, contains some caffeine, which can make sensitive individuals feel a little hyper. So enjoy your chocolate, but don't overdo.

Peanut Butter

"It sticks to your ribs," as Dennis the Menace used to say. Whether you spread it on a sandwich with slices of banana, pair it with that other epicurean classic, grape jelly, serve it on celery stalks as an appetizer or just dig into a jar with a spoon, peanut butter is an incomparable comfort food. Yes, it's full of fat, but it's the type of fat that can actually reduce your risk for heart disease. I still wouldn't dig in and eat half a jar, but small amounts can give your health a boost, and if you're a peanut-butter fan, it can add real quality to your life. Peanut butter also:

- **Provides you with vitamin E.** Recent research has suggested that vitamin E in supplement form may not be so good for you, and some scientists are now suggesting you get your daily requirements from food only. The U.S. Department of Agriculture has compiled data that show peanut butter ranks among the top-ten sources of vitamin E in the American diet.
- **Offers great all-around nutrition.** In addition to vitamin E, the peanuts in peanut butter are a rich source of monosaturated fatty acids, magnesium, folate, copper, arginine and fiber. Every one of these nutrients can help reduce your risk for circulatory and heart disease. It's also a good source of protein. Two level tablespoons provide the same amount of high-quality protein as one ounce of meat.
- **Makes you feel full.** Researchers at Purdue University demonstrated that even when they added 500 extra calories worth of peanuts or peanut butter a day to the diets of test subjects, nobody gained weight. Why? People feel full more quickly when eating peanuts, and as a result, they consume less food in their diet.
- **Lowers your triglyceride level.** Triglycerides are fatty substances (lipids) in the blood, and like cholesterol, they can raise your risk of heart disease. The same study at Purdue showed that eating peanuts can lower triglyceride levels by as much as 24 percent.

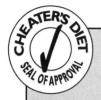

SMUCKER'S PEANUT BUTTER

By law, peanut butter must be composed of at least 90 percent peanuts. The remaining 10 percent can be a deal breaker, however, when it comes to choosing a brand. Large commercial producers generally keep the peanut content at about 94 percent, but sometimes add sugar to sweeten the taste. Although you're free to eat sugar on the weekends, it really does represent empty calories, and you may not want sugary peanut butter sticking to your teeth. Many national brands also contain trans-fatty acids (partially hydrogenated vegetable oils), which aren't great for your health. Many gourmet brands, made only with nuts, are available in specialty stores, but your local supermarket probably carries Smucker's All-Natural peanut butters, which are made from nuts and salt only. Smucker's also has a salt-free version for people who are worried about high blood pressure. You can also find some wonderful organic peanut butters at health-food stores and co-ops.

Peanut butter, which contains about 200 calories per tablespoon, is a much more concentrated food than an equal amount of fresh peanuts. That's why the Cheater's Diet allows peanuts on weekdays, but peanut butter only on weekends. And remember, even "good" fats are bad if you consume too much of them, so don't go overboard with peanut butter, even on Saturdays and Sundays. Limiting yourself to two level tablespoons a day is probably a good idea.

Cinnamon Buns

Okay, calling cinnamon buns health food may be a bit of a stretch. They do contain a lot of calories in the form of fat, as well as sugar and other carbohydrates. But they also contain an ingredient that is surprisingly good for you: cinnamon. Obviously, you don't want to eat cinnamon buns on a regular basis, but as a very occasional treat, why not reward yourself? Of course, you can always have your cinnamon on apple pie, a baked apple, rice pudding or those old-fashioned candy truffles called "Irish potatoes." Or if you want to get the great flavor without all the sugar and fat, add some powdered cinnamon to your coffee or tea. Here's what cinnamon can do for you:

- **Improve your blood sugar metabolism.** One study showed that taking a quarter of a teaspoon of cinnamon per day, over twenty days, then stopping for twenty days, lowered blood glucose levels in some people with type-2 diabetes by as much as 29 percent. Taking greater amounts, oddly, didn't have as positive an effect. Glucose levels lowered, but they didn't remain that way for the twenty-day rest period. By the way, I'm not recommending that you eat cinnamon buns if you have diabetes. People coping with that disease need to follow their doctor's advice.
- **Lower your triglyceride level.** Among the same group of people, taking more cinnamon led to lower, healthier levels of lipids in the blood. Subjects saw improvements ranging from 23 percent to 30 percent. Those taking the most—about 1³/₄ teaspoons a day—saw the most improvement.
- **Lower bad cholesterol.** In the same experiment, subjects

taking from 1 to 1¾ teaspoons of cinnamon a day lowered their LDL (bad cholesterol) level by 10 percent to 24 percent. Those taking only a quarter of a teaspoon didn't see any change in LDL level.

For those who don't care for the taste of cinnamon but would still like to enjoy the great health benefits of using it, cinnamon supplements in capsule form are available at your local health-food store.

CINNABON® CINNAMON BUNS

If you're going to have a cinnamon bun, you may as well go for the best: Cinnabon. These bad boys are made with a freshly baked eight-ounce sweet roll, Indonesian cinnamon, brown sugar and cream cheese. The regular-size Cinnabon contains 670 calories and 34 grams of fat, so you might want to limit your portion to half of one and your indulgence to only very occasional weekends.

Ice Cream

Like many comfort foods, ice cream is full of fat and sugar, but unlike many, you can reduce the damage by substituting one of the delectable low-fat, low-carb varieties at your local supermarket. You can also combine ice cream with other "health" foods mentioned here, such as nuts and chocolate. Eating ice cream, however, offers nutritious, healthful benefits all on its own. Don't believe it? Here's what ice cream does for you:

- **Provides you with calcium.** One cup of ice cream offers about 300 mg of calcium, or the equivalent of an eight-ounce glass of whole milk. If you're eating premium brands, like Häagan-Dazs, don't eat more than half a cup a day. If you go for a low-fat, low-carb substitute, however, a whole cup is entirely reasonable. By the way, calcium does more than strengthen your bones. It influences the agouti gene, which helps determine whether food that's eaten is burned as fuel or stored as fat. People who have higher calcium intake tend to burn more of their food as fuel—and so tend to be thinner.

- **Improves calcium absorption.** Choosing low-fat ice cream offers a benefit you may not be aware of: It contains a highly soluble fiber called inulin. Inulin is used to give the ice cream a smooth consistency, but experiments have shown that eating it actually increases calcium absorption. This is especially important for adolescent girls, who experience their greatest need for and ability to absorb calcium during their teenage years, but tend not to get nearly enough—often because they're dieting. If they don't get enough calcium at this time in their lives, their risk for osteoporosis in later years goes way up.

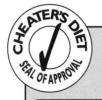

HEALTHY CHOICE ICE CREAM

Lots of ice cream makers offer excellent low-fat varieties, but my preference and personal favorites are Healthy Choice ice creams. Over the years, I've recommended Healthy Choice products to my patients in all food categories. They're consistently high in quality and taste. To double the health benefit of Healthy Choice ice creams, try Chocolate Chocolate Chunk. You'll get the taste and antioxidants of chocolate along with the calcium of ice cream, all at only 2 grams of fat, 120 calories and 21 grams of carbs per serving.

Strawberry Shortcake

Is there any dessert more wonderful on a warm spring day than ripe, ruby-red strawberries embedded in a mountain of whipped cream sitting on an island of moist, sweet biscuit? Early American settlers created the first strawberry shortcakes in imitation of a strawberry bread made by native Americans. Today, it's a staple among confections around the world. Use fresh strawberries, of course, and you can bake your own shortcake or use a commercial brand. If you buy it, check that there's nothing among the first three label ingredients containing the words "partially hydrogenated." That signals transfatty acids, which are not particularly healthful for you.

Making your own whipped cream is easy, and you'll know exactly what's in it. Just whip a half cup of ice-cold whipping cream with a half teaspoon of Splenda, and add a dash of vanilla flavoring.

The whipped cream and cake aren't health foods, it's true, but strawberries, on the other hand, taste great and:

- **Lower blood pressure.** Studies show that people who eat one serving of strawberries (eight berries) a day show significant decreases in their systolic blood pressure—that's the top number in 120/80. This suggests that strawberries may help ward off heart disease associated with hypertension.
- **Raise folate levels.** Folate, or folic acid, is an important nutrient that helps to lower homocysteine levels in the blood. Homocysteine is an amino acid that can cause arteries to close up.
- **Add fiber to your diet.** One cup of strawberries contains four grams of dietary fiber, which is good news for your heart and intestines. Fiber also helps prevent high blood sugar, keeps HDL (good) cholesterol levels high, lowers triglycerides (particles that carry fat in the bloodstream), prevents apple-shape obesity and reduces the risk of certain cancers.
- **Shower you with antioxidants.** Strawberries are among the very best sources of antioxidants known, especially of a type called anthocyanins, which give the fruit its red color. Antioxidants are your body's powerful fighters of cancer and heart disease. Just because a food contains high concentrations of antioxidants, however, doesn't

mean the body will absorb them. In the case of straw-berries, research has shown that the body's level of antioxidants peaks markedly within thirty to sixty min-utes after eating them, a sure sign that nearly complete absorption has taken place.

Cheese

You can cook with cheese or serve it on its own as an appe-tizer, snack or part of a healthful meal. You can add it to sand-wiches, sprinkle it on pasta or serve it—perhaps with a drop of aged balsamic vinegar—as a dessert. It is a wonderful accompaniment to a glass of wine. And it is full of fat, fat, fat. A single ounce of cheddar contains about six grams of satu-rated fat—about one-third your daily allowance. So you can't have it every day, but on the weekends, why not? The fact is, cheese offers some great health benefits if you eat it in mod-eration—a couple of ounces, cut into small pieces, is plenty, and it's enough to let cheese work its magic, as it:

- **Helps keep your teeth healthy.** Some research has sug-gested that eating hard cheese along with or after eating foods that contain carbohydrates can help counter the acid attacks launched against your teeth by plaque bacteria.
- **Lets you absorb nutrients.** Remember that lycopene you get from eating pizza? You can only absorb it in the pres-ence of fat, which is why the cheese on pizza is so impor-tant. You also need fat to absorb alpha- and beta-carotenes, nutrients that help prevent cancer and heart disease.
- **Provides calcium.** Cheese is a great source of calcium. Experts now recommend that older people consume at

least 1,200 milligrams of calcium a day, and kids aged 9 through 18 consume at least 1,300.

- **Protects against breast cancer.** One study suggested that high levels of a nutrient called conjugated linoleic acid, found in cheese and other dairy products, can reduce the number and incidence of breast tumors. Conjugated linoleic acid in high doses has also been shown to help people lose weight, but the concentration in milk fat isn't high enough to have that effect.

Breads

If you've been following a low-carb diet, whichever weight-loss guru invented it has probably told you that the love of bread, not money, is the root of all evil. Well, it's true that we love it. When we deny ourselves the pleasure of having some now and then, we may even get a little grumpy craving it. So have some. Why not? It's the weekend, and for heaven's sake, whatever you've been told about the terrible health effects of carbohydrates, a slice of rye is not the nutritional equivalent of a cigarette. There are reasons bread has been called the "staff of life." While processed white bread can indeed make you fat, rye, whole-grain and many pumpernickel varieties are full of healthful fiber and vitamins. Some research has shown that eating these breads in moderation can help you live longer.

When you buy bread, look for the word "whole" on the package. You can also look for the "Whole Grain Stamp," an official packaging symbol created by the Whole Grains Council, which tells you the product is an "excellent" (full serving of whole grain) or a "good" (half serving of whole grain) source of grain.

Need more evidence? Consider that bread can also:

- **Prevent heart disease.** Two studies at Harvard, one of 40,000 male health professionals and a similar one of female nurses, showed about a 40 percent decrease in risk for heart disease among people who consumed a lot of fiber. This was especially true for cereal fiber, the type found in bread. Several studies also suggested that a high fiber intake can help ward off metabolic syndrome—a constellation of diseases and symptoms that includes fat accumulation around the middle of the body, type-2 diabetes, elevated blood pressure, low HDL (good) cholesterol and high triglycerides, which are particles that carry fat in the bloodstream.

- **Improve bowel health.** High fiber intake can help prevent diverticular disease, an inflammation of the large bowel that can become very painful. More and more people face this condition as they get older—one-third of people over forty-five and half of everyone over eighty-five have it. Likewise, eating more bread can help prevent and relieve constipation, the most common digestive complaint in the United States. One caution: Whenever you increase your fiber intake, you should also drink more fluids, as the fiber absorbs water and will carry a lot out of your system.

- **Fight hormone-related cancers.** Early research suggested that whole grains could prevent bowel cancer. Those results have become controversial, as later studies didn't support them. However, whole grain has been shown to lower the risk of hormone-related cancers, a group which includes tumors of the breast, uterus and prostate, by 10 to 40 percent.

Meat

If you're following a low- to moderate-fat diet during the week, you probably find yourself craving a sirloin steak or pork chop every now and then. (If you're on a high-protein, low-carb diet, you're probably craving everything else in this list.) You have probably heard that beef is bad for you, and pork is worse. Well, listen up. Over the past three decades, the meat industry has worked hard to lower the fat and cholesterol in their products. Today's lean cuts of beef and pork often contain less fat than a skinless chicken leg. Both types of meat can be a significant source of nutrition when eaten in moderate amounts—say an eight-ounce cut, broiled, at a restaurant on a Friday night, or a juicy, plump hamburger cooked on the grill on a Saturday afternoon. By the way, pork loin, which is extremely lean, can become part of your diet even on weekdays. What else can meat do for you?

- **Beef gives you Bs.** A three-ounce serving of beef gives you 75 percent of your daily requirement for vitamin B_{12}, which you need to keep your red blood cells healthy, as well as to metabolize fats, proteins and carbohydrates.
- **Meat offers iron.** Both beef and pork are good sources of iron. The type of iron they contain is called heme iron, which is much easier to absorb than other types. This is especially important for women, as iron deficiency is a common problem for them. You need iron to manufacture hemoglobin in your blood. You also need it to metabolize all those B vitamins you're getting from your beef.
- **Grass-fed beef has omega-3s.** That's right. You may have thought that you could only find these healthful oils in

salmon and flaxseed, but cows that have been raised eating range grass instead of grain cattle feed contain substantial levels of omega-3 fatty acids. That's good news for your heart!

- **Pork is like nature's own vitamin pill.** It contains magnesium, phosphorous, potassium, zinc, thiamin, riboflavin (it's one of the best sources known for this vitamin), niacin, B_{12} and B_6.

- **Meat means high-quality protein.** When you think protein, meat is the standard against which all other sources are measured. Any kind of meat provides about seven grams of protein per ounce. Protein is used for building and repairing muscle and other tissues, red blood cells, hair and fingernails. It's also used to make hormones. In short, you can't live without protein, and meat is a great source.

Nuts

Nuts grow on trees. Peanuts, which grow in the ground, are legumes and aren't part of the nut family. Although peanuts have many healthful properties, here we're talking about almonds, pecans, Brazil nuts, hazelnuts, walnuts, chestnuts, cashews and anything else that has a shell, is edible, hangs from a branch and gets 75 percent of its calories from fat. Now, you might ask, "How can something that gets most of its calories from fat be healthful?" Most of the fats are monosaturated and polyunsaturated, which means they won't raise your cholesterol level. Now, do yourself a favor. Salt can raise blood pressure in certain people, so when you buy shelled or packaged nuts, choose ones that haven't been drenched in salt or oil. Do that, and you'll truly reap the health benefits of nuts, such as:

- **Loads of vitamins and minerals.** Nuts are good sources of niacin, thiamin, folate, selenium, copper, phosphorus, magnesium and manganese, and they're a lot tastier than your average multivitamin.
- **Protection from radical damage.** Nuts are rich in antioxidants, so like any other food that offers this benefit, they help protect you from free-radical damage that contributes to the onset of cancer and heart disease.
- **High protein.** Nuts are one of the best sources in the plant world for protein. An ounce of nuts gives you the same amount of protein as an equal amount of beef.
- **Lower cholesterol.** Researchers in Toronto found that people who ate two handfuls of almonds a day for one month reduced their LDL (bad) cholesterol by 12 percent, relative to their levels of HDL (good) cholesterol. Eating one handful a day reduced LDL by 7.8 percent. Be careful, though. Two handfuls is a lot of nuts—about 500 calories. For weight-loss purposes, eat them on weekends only, and make sure you take their high caloric value into consideration.

In chapter 4, I note that peanuts are allowed Monday through Friday, while other nuts aren't. That's because research has shown that peanuts actually help curb your appetite, and when you eat them, you cut calories in other parts of your diet without even thinking about it. Tree nuts don't have that effect, and it can be very difficult to stop after one handful. So save the macadamias for the weekends. And when you do have some nuts, they might go great with an ice-cold glass of . . .

Beer

For some of you, it may seem as if I've saved the best for last. We see a lot in the media about the positive health effects of wine, but what do we hear about beer? That it gives you a big belly. Of course, if you guzzle it down by the six-pack every day, it *will* make you fat. But if you have a bottle or two on a Saturday and Sunday afternoon, sports fans, it may just end up being a lifesaver for you, because beer helps:

- **Preserve your eyesight.** Beer, especially darker varieties such as ale and stout, has recently been shown in labora-tory tests to reduce the incidence of cataracts. Anti-oxidants in beer protect cells in the eye and have proven particularly beneficial to people with diabetes.
- **Lower your risk for heart disease.** A laboratory study at the University of Scranton showed that drinking two beers a day may halve your risk for atherosclerosis—the buildup of plaque in the walls of your arteries. Two beers every day can add a significant calorie load to your daily intake, so I wouldn't recommend daily drinking based on this study alone. But on the weekends, why not?
- **Cut your risk for cancer.** A laboratory study in Japan suggested that compounds in beer might fight cancer. Lab animals that drank beer instead of water reduced DNA damage in their lungs, liver and kidneys by 85 percent. Unfortunately, the study used only non-alcohol beer, so there's no way to say for sure whether beer with alcohol has the same effect in people.

As with wine—or any binge food—if you have a problem with alcohol, skip the beer, even the non-alcohol kind. I've heard far too many tales about people starting with "near-beer" and then moving on to the real thing.

Of course, the cheat foods mentioned in this chapter are just the beginning of the types of foods you can cheat with on the weekends. I've tried to stick to healthful recommendations, with the possible exception of cinnamon buns—ah, well, nobody's perfect. The important things to remember when choosing your cheat foods are to avoid binge foods and to be reasonable in the amounts of sugar and fat you consume. No matter which foods you choose, remember that you're cheating, so enjoy!

FIFTY (TRULY) GUILT-FREE CHEAT FOODS

Archway Chocolate Chip Drop Cookies

Archway Coconut Macaroons

Archway Peanut Jumble Cookies

Archway Pecan Icebox Cookies

Bacon

Bagel chips

Barbara's Bakery Animal Cookies

Barbara's Bakery Crisp Cookies

Barbara's Bakery Snackimals

Beef jerky

Borden Twin Pops

Bran breads

Breyer's Vanilla Frozen Yogurt

Croutons

Dolly Madison Gem Variety Donuts

Dolly Madison Powdered Mini Donuts

Entenmann's Soft Baked Cookies

Eskimo Pie Fudge Bar

Famous Amos Butter Shorties

Famous Amos Chocolate Chip Cookies

Famous Amos Pecan Shorties

Frito-Lay Beef Sticks

Dole Fruit Juice Bars (no sugar added)

Fudgesicles

Ham

Healthy Choice Corned Beef

Healthy Choice Popcorn

Hebrew National Corned Beef

Honey Maid Grahams (all types)

Hood Fat-Free Egg Nog

Hostess Donettes

Ice Cream

Jell-O Pop Bars

Jell-O Pudding Bars

Keebler Classic Collection Cookies

Keebler Club Crackers

Keebler Townhouse Crackers

Kellogg's Rice Krispies

Kellogg's Rice Krispies Caramel/Peanut Butter Treats

Kellogg's Rice Krispies Double Chocolate Chunk Treats

Kellogg's Rice Krispies Original Treat Bar

Kellogg's Rice Krispies Scotcheroos

Frostick Juice Flavored Sticks

Kool-Aid Pops

Manischewitz Biscotti

Manischewitz Chocolate Macaroons

Manischewitz Matzo Crackers

Microwave popcorn (most brands)

Milky Way Snack Bar (juice bar)

Nabisco Better Cheddars crackers

Nabisco Chocolate Snaps

Nabisco Chocolate Wafers

Nabisco Nilla Wafers

Nabisco Teddy Graham Snacks (all types)

Nabisco Triscuit Wafers

Nestlé IceScreamers Shock Tarts

Nestlé IceScreamers Tiger Tails

Panda Licorice Chews

Pastrami

Pepperidge Farm Distinctive Cookies: Bordeaux, Pirouette, Brussels, Mint Brussels, Mint Milano, Chantilly Hazelnut Raspberry, Chessman, Toy Chest Butter, Double Chocolate Milano

Pepperidge Farm Old Fashioned Cookies (all types)

Rice cakes (These don't seem like a cheat food, but if you've ever been on a carb-free diet, you know why this is included.)

Ritz Stoneground/Wheatsworth Crackers

Sausage

Scrapple

Smart Pop Low Fat Popcorn

Snackwell's Chocolate Chip Cookies

Starburst Juice Bars

Stella D'oro Angel Bars

Stella D'oro Castellettes

Stella D'oro Egg Biscuits

Stella D'oro Egg Jumbo

Stella D'oro Swiss Fudge

Swiss Miss Cocoa Diet Cocoa Mix

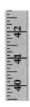

Swiss Miss Cocoa Fat Free

Switzer Licorice Bites

Three Musketeers Snack Bars

Weight Watchers Smart Ones Chocolate Mousse

Welch's Tropical Coolers (fruit juice bar)

4

The Do's and Don'ts of Weekday Weight Loss

I am a doctor, so I want you to live well, not die thin. Patients often ask me if cheating on the weekends will work with low-fat, low-carb, grapefruit or other diets. The short answer is yes, but that doesn't mean I believe most of the fad diets out there are good for you. It's never made much sense to me to put people on an unhealthful diet, no matter how effectively it takes off the pounds.

So far as I'm concerned, the best weekday diet you can follow is one structured around whole foods, specifically fresh fruits and vegetables, whole grains, legumes and cold-water fish, with some pork loin thrown in now and then for taste. It should also offer variety, both because eating from a broad array of foods works against boredom and because doing so may be even more important to maintaining your health than simply cutting out foods that aren't all that good for you.

One recent study looked at the dietary habits of five thousand French men and women and found that they consumed more foods that were higher in total fat, saturated fat and cholesterol than Americans did. In fact, nearly all of the French women derived more than 10 percent of their calories from saturated fat, yet on average they were far thinner than their American counterparts and had a lower incidence of heart disease. What makes the difference is the variety in their diets. The results suggest to me that what you put on your plate is even more important than what you leave off of it.

Cheating with Other Diets

Eating from a wide variety of choices, including lots of healthful ones, is difficult in a culture that constantly tempts you with fried food and sugar everywhere you turn. Sometimes, denying yourself a whole class of foods seems easier than trying to limit yourself to moderate consumption, in the same way that habitual drinkers completely avoid alcohol. Thus we find ourselves standing in awe at the immense popularity of low- and no-carb diets, and before them, low- and no-fat diets.

Though the relative health advantages of these diets have been hotly debated, there's no doubt that both work to lower weight. In fact, two recent studies reviewed by Harvard

University's Health Newsletter demonstrated conclusively that after a year, dieters on both types of diet fare equally well in terms of total weight loss. And if you happen to be following one of them now, you should see continued—and probably increased—weight loss if you cheat on the weekends.

Although you can lose weight following either a low-fat or low-carb diet, why would you do such a thing? The fact is, you can't live completely without either carbohydrates or fats because your body needs them in order to function. They are not your enemies, and trying to eliminate either from your diet completely will leave you with an incredibly monotonous menu plan.

The Cheater's Diet recognizes that there are some principles from both types of diets that you would be wise to follow. Specifically, you should eat less sugar, syrup, white flour and partially hydrogenated oil. You can eat some of these items over the weekends (although I strongly recommend that you get the partially hydrogenated stuff out of your life altogether), but on the weekdays, you need to be very strict with yourself about them. Remember to read labels. If you see corn syrup, fructose or hydrogenated among the ingredients, put the item down and make another choice.

Other than that, three rules must apply to every morsel you put into your mouth during the work week: It's got to be nutritious, it's got to be delicious, and it's got to help you lose weight. Beyond those basics, you'll eat three meals a day, consisting mostly of whole foods, with small snacks allowed in between. I know that many diet plans tell you to eat five or six smaller meals a day, which will help keep your blood sugar level steady and curb your appetite. For most people, however, taking so much time out to eat is simply not realistic, especially if you have a day job or a tribe of kids. Plan on three meals a day, and you can grab a snack on the run if you start to feel hungry.

Portion Control Made Simple

Portion control is important. There are a couple of ways to keep your intake within reasonable limits without actually counting calories. The first is simply to divide up your plate into quarters: one for proteins; one for veggies or fruits; and one for complex carbs, like whole-grain and semolina pasta, yams, lentils, legumes, brown rice, vegetables and wheat germ. You can live without bread, white rice and white potatoes during the week. The carbohydrates will give you an energy boost, but if you've reached your fourth decade, your body may no longer be able to burn all that extra fuel, so you should feel free to substitute another helping of vegetables instead. Either leave the last quarter of your plate empty or fill it with veggies. (Can you tell I'm big on vegetables?)

The other way to measure portions at a glance is to compare them to familiar objects. One portion (1 cup) of cooked vegetables is the size of your fist. A medium fruit is as big as a baseball. A single portion (½ cup) of pasta, rice or potatoes is the same size as a strictly measured scoop of ice cream. One serving of protein (3 ounces) is the size of a deck of cards or the palm of your hand. (Basketball players obviously get a break on that last one.)

There are some simple do's and don'ts that will keep your meals low in starches and saturated (bad) fats, while high in fiber and the good monosaturated, polyunsaturated and omega-3 fats, as well as healthful carbs and lean proteins.

The Don'ts

There are some foods that you must avoid during the workweek:

- **Sugar.** It looks so pure and innocent, and it tastes so good. But there are no two ways about it: Eating sugar—whether it's table sugar (sucrose), corn sugar (fructose) or honey— makes you gain weight. Not only does some of it go straight to your belly, butt and thighs, but the body uses the rest as fuel instead of drawing on your stores of fat. As if that weren't enough, through a series of complex reactions in the body and brain, consuming sugar also increases hunger and thirst. This is especially true of sugary drinks, including fruit drinks and juices. Soda pop is the worst, and colas are the worst of the worst. So avoid them. Obviously, also avoid cookies, cakes, donuts and candy. Read labels on packaged goods. If one of the ingredients is corn syrup, don't eat it. In fact, so many different forms of sugar are added to processed foods that it's best to avoid the issue altogether and eat fresh, whole produce when you can.
- **Bread.** Bread, especially white, expands your waistline. Sorry. I know you didn't want to hear that. If you've been on a low-carb diet, you miss eating bread. You may even yearn for it. Unfortunately, it breaks down fast in your gut, then turns into sugar and is stored as fat very easily. A Tufts University study of 459 men and women showed that those who ate the most white bread had an increase in waist measurement five times greater than those who ate the least. There is some good news, however. Whole-grain breads

are delicious and good for you, so you're certainly allowed to eat them—on the weekends. Most commercial brands contain some sugar, so make sure that it's listed way down in the ingredient list. Oh, and don't try to get away with eating pretzels, muffins, bagels or baked desserts on the weekdays. You know better.

ABS: YOUR WEIGHT'S BIGGEST ENEMIES

Think of the acronym "ABS."

A is for Alcohol. Stick with drinking alcohol on Saturday and Sunday only, and limit yourself to one or two glasses of wine. While there is evidence that moderate, daily consumption of wine or beer has health benefits, if you're overweight, burning off fat is even more healthful. Drinking alcohol of any kind during the workweek will make losing weight that much harder to do.

B is for Breads. Again, breads of all kinds seem to encourage weight gain. If you have a craving for bread during the week, substitute whole-wheat tortillas.

S is for Sugars. Sugar makes you fat. It doesn't matter whether it's table sugar, corn syrup or fructose, which is also made from corn. Read the last three letters of each ingredient on a package. Any word that ends in "ose" is a sugar. Soda and fruit drinks are among the worst offenders.

• **Saturated Fats.** Some very popular diets let you eat all the fat you want. There is also a lot of overwhelming evidence that diets high in saturated fat lead to heart disease, cancers and strokes, the three most common killers in America. Some people are willing to take that risk because—thanks to all those diet gurus out there—they seem to believe that eating saturated fat is necessary in order to lose weight. Well, to use a saturated metaphor, that's a bunch of baloney. The argument is that these fatty foods give a more prolonged sense of fullness, which is true. But the same effect can be achieved with the good fats I'll recommend later. By the way, saturated fats, which are present in red meat, hard cheeses, butter and lard, are not the only "bad" fats. That list also includes hydrogenated and partially hydrogenated oils. Skip foods that list the word "hydrogenated" anywhere in the first three ingredients on the label. Specifically, during the workweek avoid butter, palm oil, fatty beef (not sirloin), cheese that's not skim, fast foods, fried chicken, fried fish, fried desserts, French fries, muffins, crackers, microwave popcorn (if it contains bad fats or oils) and coffee that contains cream. In fact, you're better off not eating that stuff at all, so try to resist. Donuts, cookies, cakes, pies and the like offer a double threat: They're full of saturated fat *and* sugar. Oh, and remember, not all trans fats and saturated fats come from animal products. Some also come from plants, so don't be fooled by fast-food restaurants' claims that their products are more healthful because they cook with vegetable oil. You weren't born yesterday.

• **Alcohol.** There are clearly some health benefits of moderate alcohol intake, but weight loss isn't one of them. Beer, wine and spirits are relatively high in calories, but there's a bigger problem: Alcohol is burned preferentially by the body. In other words, when you eat and drink, you'll use the alcohol for fuel and store the food, in the same way you do with sugar. Also, like sugar, alcohol can make you feel hungry, and many people associate it psychologically with junk foods like chips and pretzels. My advice? Save it for the weekend.

FEWER CALORIES, LONGER LIFE?

For a long time, scientists have suspected that cutting daily calorie food consumption by one-third (to about 1,500) would slow down the aging process and extend the average human life span. It works that way for yeast cells, worms, fruit flies and, more recently, primates—which may be very good news for us humans, especially those who have already adopted caloric restriction as a way of life. Among other benefits, it seems to reduce and even reverse cellular damage due to aging, protect against certain cancers and help regulate insulin levels.

Properly balanced nutrition, however, is an extremely important consideration for anyone who is cutting calories so drastically. If this lifestyle interests you and you'd like to try it, you'll first need to transform your daily diet to a healthful one that includes plenty of fresh fruits, vegetables and whole grains. You can add fish a couple of times a week and very lean pork loin for an occasional treat. Once you've lived on this diet for six months, you can gradually begin reducing the amount of food you eat each day. Be aware, however, that this is not a choice that allows for cheating, and it's more for health than weight loss.

The Do's

Enough with the don'ts. Let's talk about the foods you *can* eat. It's more fun.

- **Protein.** You should have at least three servings of protein a day. There is no upper limit, as you'll find your body won't want any more when you've had enough. That is, your appetite will go away. Proteins are used to build and repair body tissue as well as keep your metabolism functioning properly. They're also great for controlling food cravings. Many of my patients complain about late-afternoon cravings when they haven't had proteins at lunch. The same holds true for their evenings after a protein-less dinner. And I suspect that a protein snack at night would help prevent cravings throughout the wee hours. High-quality proteins, such as those listed at the end of this paragraph, are best. They contain the amino acid leucine, which is necessary for appetite control and metabolism. In their quest to eat healthful foods, many of my patients chronically get too little protein, but I urge them and you to do otherwise. Here are some top sources of protein:
  - Black beans
  - Chicken
  - Clams
  - Cod
  - Crab
  - Fresh eggs
  - Haddock
  - Lobster

- Low fat cheeses
- Low-fat dairy
- Mahi-mahi
- Peanuts
- Pinto beans
- Pork loin
- Red kidney beans
- Salmon
- Sardines
- Scallops
- Shrimp
- Sirloin
- Skim milk
- Small red beans
- Sole
- Tilapia (St. Peter's fish)
- Tuna
- Turkey
- Turkey bacon
- Turkey sausage

- **Salmon, Tuna and Sardines.** These foods are rich in the good fats that help prevent heart disease. Get fresh (not farm-raised) salmon, and avoid albacore tuna, which is higher in mercury content.

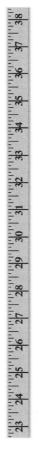

FOUR-STAR FOODS:
THE BEST OF THE BEST

Try to include at least one of these foods in your diet every day.

Bell peppers

Berries (any type)

Broccoli (cooked or raw)

Canned salmon (pink or sockeye)

Garlic

Kale

Onions (raw)

Progresso Pizza Sauce

Salmon (Atlantic, Chinook, sockeye)

Spinach (cooked)

Tomato (cherry)

Tomato (med slice)

Tomato ketchup

Tomato puree

Tomato salsa

Tomato sauce

Wheat germ

• **Chicken Breast and Turkey Breast.** Without the skin, these are your best and leanest poultry choices. And speaking of poultry, eggs are also great food. They have a bad reputation because their yolks contain a lot of cholesterol, but there's no good evidence that eating eggs raises the cholesterol level in your blood. You can have an egg or two every day. While you should skip the bacon and pork or beef sausage, turkey substitutes will please your palate and contain less fat.

- **Peanuts.** They're great for snacks, but limit them to a handful a day. They contain healthful fat and, in fact, promote weight loss.

- **Yogurt.** Go for the nonfat, plain varieties. You can add a sugar substitute and/or fresh fruit if you prefer a sweeter taste. Some research has suggested that eating three servings of low-fat yogurt a day can increase your weight loss by as much as 22 percent, and the associated fat loss seems to take place mostly in the trunk region. The same rule applies for all other dairy foods, which are high in protein: Go nonfat.

- **Fruits and Vegetables.** One of the hallmarks of a healthful diet is the inclusion of lots of fruits and vegetables. Plant produce is bursting with nutrients like vitamins, minerals and phytochemicals, as well as some healthful fats, while generally containing few calories. Dark-green, leafy vegetables are often cited as being the most healthful, but the fact is that any veggie that has a brilliant color—red, yellow, orange, purple, green, you name it— is telling you to come and get it. It's in these very colors that most of a food's antioxidants are contained.

THE SALAD STRATEGY

Have a salad that includes tuna, salmon or chicken, and low-fat mozzarella and low-fat dressing twenty minutes before a meal. It will cut your appetite for the main course and help you feel satisfied longer. Tomato is the best vegetable there is. Lycopene is associated with significantly lowered risk for many kinds of cancer. This is one vegetable that's best eaten with some fat for absorption. Try it with some mozzarella slices and sprinkled with olive oil.

It's a good idea to have a fruit or vegetable serving every two or three hours. Doing this instead of munching on junk food can give you a one-pound-per-week weight loss in and of itself. Following is a list of some of the most nutritious fruits and vegetables.

- Applesauce (unsweetened)
- Apples (Gala, Granny Smith, red)
- Blueberries
- Cherries
- Grapefruit
- Lemons
- Oranges
- Plums
- Pomegranates
- Raspberries
- Strawberries
- Tangerines
- Watermelon
- Artichokes
- Asparagus
- Avocado
- Bell peppers
- Broccoli
- Broccoli sprouts
- Brussels sprouts
- Cabbage
- Carrots
- Cauliflower
- Celery
- Chard

- Collard greens
- Dandelions
- Eggplant
- Horseradish
- Jalapeños
- Kale
- Lettuce
- Mushrooms
- Mustard greens
- Onions
- Peas
- Radishes
- Spinach
- Tomato
- Yams and sweet potatoes
- Zucchini

You should have at least three servings of fruit a day. By the way, apples, which are very high in fiber, can be a real ally where fighting fat is concerned. Eating a small to medium apple about a half hour before every meal helps cut your appetite and enhances weight loss. Studies show that eating grapefruit three times a day can also lead to significant weight loss—but I certainly am not endorsing the old grapefruit fad diet, which is not healthful. I'm saying that eating grapefruit as part of a health-promoting diet is a good idea.

Berries, prunes, plums and apples are all high in chemicals that fight heart disease and cancer. Smoothies with fresh fruit, as well as nonfat yogurt with sugar substitutes are also great for snacks. Fresh and frozen fruits are best, but you can have canned fruit if it has no added sugar. For fruit juice, squeeze your own and sweeten it with a sugar substitute.

A few fruits are best left for the weekend, as their sugar content is quite high. These include pineapples, bananas, cantaloupes and grapes.

Vegetables are good fresh, frozen or canned. Steaming is a great way to prepare them. A very healthful approach is to sprinkle your vegetables with some olive oil and Morton's Lite Salt, a great salt substitute that's high in potassium. Leave corn for the weekend. Remember, corn syrup and fructose, two types of pure sugar, both come from corn.

You should have at least four servings of veggies a day— more if you like. You can eat them between meals, or you can double up your veggie portion on that empty quarter of your plate if you don't want to give up your carbohydrate portion.

Make fruits and veggies a part of your lifestyle, not just your diet. Sweet potatoes and yams are great. Pasta with tomato sauce is low in fat and a great cancer fighter. Don't worry about pasta as a carb. Semolina wheat flour isn't converted to fat in the same way that the white flour in bread is. So go back to enjoying your pasta with olive oil and tomato sauce—but remember, your serving should fill no more than one quarter of your plate.

THE PERFECT MEAL

What constitutes a "perfect" meal? A low-carb person claims one thing, a low-fat guru another. Some scientists in the Netherlands, however, recently looked at what research data predicted would be the very best meal for cardiovascular health. They called it the "polymeal." It contains red wine, cold-water fish such as salmon or tuna, dark chocolate, fruits, vegetables, garlic and almonds. Estimates are that if you eat this kind of fare every day (fish two to four times per week), you'll reduce your risk for heart disease by more than 75 percent. To lose weight, I recommend you save the wine, chocolate and almonds for the weekends, but the rest of the diet is perfect for weekdays.

• **Fats.** Not all fats are created equal. Some are good, but in excess, some are not so good. Confused? A lot of people are. Here's the deal: The not-so-good fats, which come from animal products such as meat, butter and lard, are the saturated kinds. They turn solid at room temperature. Consuming them causes your liver to manufacture too much cholesterol, which can lead to heart disease, stroke and cancer. As far as I'm concerned, they're part of too many diet plans, and they should not be part of yours—at least Monday through Friday. You can eat them

OMEGA-3 FATTY ACIDS: CAN FAT REALLY BE GOOD FOR YOU?

Inuits (Eskimos) who still subsist on a native diet eat so much fat that you'd think they would be crippled with health problems, but they're not. In fact, they experience a lower incidence of degenerative conditions such as coronary heart disease, rheumatoid arthritis, diabetes mellitus and psoriasis than people who live on a typical Western diet. The reason seems to be that they consume a high volume of omega-3 fatty acids, which is the type of fat you find in cold-water fish, as well as seals and whales. These fats reduce inflammation, keep your blood from excessive clotting and seem particularly healthful for the heart. The body uses fats to construct the membranes of all of its cells, and omega-3s make membranes that are very elastic and pliant. Saturated fats, however, result in much stiffer membranes, which, among other effects, can make the return to a resting state more difficult for your heart. Omega-3 fatty acids come in three varieties: the types found in fish, which are called eicosapentaenoic acid (EPA) and docosahexanoic acid (DHA); and the kind found in flax seed and dark-green leafy vegetables, called alpha-linolenic acid (ALA). Although the body doesn't produce omega-3s on its own, it does have enzymes that can convert ALA to EPA.

in moderation on the weekends, because they actually can have a beneficial use—to maintain a minimum level of body fat, which you need for insulation and to fuel the body during exercise. But the good fats can do the same thing for you in a more healthful way.

Good fats are classified as either monosaturated or polyunsaturated. Monosaturated fats are liquid at room temperature, but become solid at cooler temperatures such as in your refrigerator. Polyunsaturated fats remain liquid even at very cold temperatures. Good fats, which come from plant-based foods and fish, can reduce your risk of illness and help with your body's metabolism and weight loss.

Sometimes, good fats come nicely packaged with protein, as in the case of tuna, salmon and sardines. These fish are high in a type of polyunsaturated fat called omega-3, which is great for health and weight loss. Peanuts, which are high in monosaturated fats, are also a good protein source and make an excellent snack food. Some studies show that one or two handfuls a day can contribute to weight loss.

Other good fats stand alone. The best of these is olive oil. Use olive oil in cooking, vegetables, on salads and whatever other ways you can come up with. Extra virgin, while a little more expensive, tastes best.

Olive oil is a staple of the so-called Mediterranean Diet, which is similar to the Cheater's Diet. A study at Harvard showed that women following the Mediterranean Diet lost fifteen times more weight than those following a simple low-fat diet. That's fifteen times more *while eating more fat*—but they're good fats. In the Mediterranean Diet, a whopping 38 percent of calories come from fat, but all in the form of peanuts, fish and olive oil. In addition, people on such diets are much more likely to stick with the diet.

Excess saturated fats raise the storage of body fat, especially around the belly area, and recent studies show that it also promotes the accumulation of fat around internal organs. The good fats burn off easily, reduce hunger and substitute for bad fats in the diet.

Canola is another good choice for cooking, but it is not as tasty for sprinkling. Coconut oil is also a good choice, but not the partially hydrogenated form, as its medium chain fatty acids can raise Cain with your health. DAG (diacylglycerol or diglyceride) oil, a man-made ingredient of Enova oil, is also terrific for weight loss. DAG oil is burned quickly and is not stored as fat. Patients have lost up to 48 percent more body fat eating these oils than did those who ate regular oils. Enova oil has a very neutral flavor and is good for cooking. Flaxseed oil, which contains omega-3 fatty acids, is also a great choice, but it has a strong, distinct flavor.

One caveat: You *can* have too much of a good thing. Even the good fats are, in the end, fats. Both good fats and bad fats are high in calories, and eating too much of either will work against losing weight. A piece of fish or a couple of tablespoons a day of olive oil a day is plenty—and remember, sprinkle, don't pour.

• **Snacks.** Snacks are important. They help keep your blood-sugar level even throughout the day, fight hunger and cravings, and give you the psychological satisfaction of chewing and swallowing. My first recommendation for snacks is fresh veggies or fruit. Peanuts are good as well, but no more than one or two handfuls a day. You can also indulge yourself in a nonfat fudge popsicle, sugar-free pudding, or a cup of hot cocoa made with nonfat milk and Splenda, but limit yourself to a portion of each. You can also have a protein shake (see page 117).

PUTTING IT ALL TOGETHER

Here are my recommendations for your diet during the week:

✓ Three servings of protein foods a day.

✓ Dairy protein every day (beware of cottage cheese—your body treats it like a carbohydrate).

✓ Three to seven servings of veggies and/or fruits a day (leave cantaloupes, grapes, pineapples, bananas and corn, all of which are high in sugar, for the weekends).

✓ Consume good fats, including cold-water fish.

✓ Sprinkle a little olive oil on your food.

✓ Pasta and whole-grain rice are good carbohydrate choices, as are sweet potatoes and yams. Two small servings a day are enough.

✓ Watch your snack portions!

There you have it. Have fun! *Bon appétit! Mangia!* And remember, the weekend will be here before you know it.

THREE-STAR FOODS

Here are some great, healthful choices for mealtimes. For condiments and sauces, go by portion size on the package. For sliced cheese, eat three or four slices a day. Condiments, dips and sauces—use just enough to taste. All vegetables are part of this list, and don't forget there are numerous four-star veggies. Remember to eat something from the four-star list every day, and you may eat from only that list if you prefer. For variety's sake, though, throw in some of the three-stars from time to time. Don't, however, eat any particular food from the three-star fare day after day. Mix it up, as there are plenty to choose from.

Eggs

Eggs (fresh)
Fleischman's Egg Beaters

Meats

Beerwurst luncheon meat (beef)
Beerwurst luncheon meat (pork)
Healthy Choice bologna
Healthy Choice smoked sausage

Dairy & Non-Dairy Substitutes

Alpine Lace Fat -Free American Cheese
Alpine Lace Fat-Free Cream Cheese
Butter Buds
Fat-free milk
Healthy Choice Fat-Free American Cheese
Healthy Choice Fat-Free Mozzarella
Kraft Deluxe Grated American Cheese
Kraft Free Singles—American Cheese
Kraft Miracle Whip Free
Kraft Miracle Whip Light
Light n' Lively Yogurt, fat-free
Molly McButter
Philadelphia Brand Fat-Free Cream Cheese
Powder Coffee-Mate, fat-free or light
Rich's Coffee Rich (non-dairy creamer) Lite
Rich's Farm Rich (non-dairy creamer) Lite/Fat Free
Ricotta (whole milk, part skim, light/low-fat)

Silk (White Wave) Creamer
Smart Beat Light American Cheese
String cheese (all brands)
Watkins Butter Sprinkles
Weight Watchers American Cheese
Weight Watchers Fat-Free Mayonnaise
Weight Watchers Swiss

Poultry

Butterball Fat-Free Turkey Breast
Chicken breast (skinless)
Chicken slices (white meat)
Healthy Choice Turkey Butterball
Smoked sausage
Turkey breast (skinless)
Turkey ham
Turkey loaf
Turkey pastrami
Turkey roll

Fish

Albacore
Herring
Mackerel
Orange roughy
Sardines
Sardines, canned (drain oil or choose without oil)
Trout
Tuna
Tuna, canned, chunk solid or white, in water or oil (drain)
Van De Kamp's Crisp and Healthy (frozen-fish filet)
Whitefish

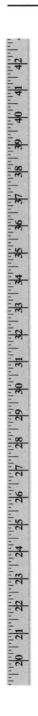

Soups/Broths

Manischewitz Borscht Low Calorie
Progresso Chicken Noodle Soup
Swanson's Beef Broth
Swanson's Chicken Broth
Swanson's Vegetable Broth

Condiments

All herbs, spices, seasonings and flavorings
Cooking sprays, all brands
Dill pickles
French's Honey Mustard
Heinz Chili Sauce
Heinz or A-1 Steak Sauce
Ketchup
Mustard
Pickle relish, 1 tablespoon
Pizza sauce, canned
Soy sauce
Taco sauce
Worcestershire sauce

Dips, Sauces and Dressings

Amy's Marinara pasta sauce
Barilla Arrabbiata pasta sauce
Classico Mushroom and Olive pasta sauce
Classico Spicy Red Pepper pasta sauce
Del Monte salsa
Hain No-Oil Range salad dressings
Healthy Choice Mushroom Alfredo pasta sauce
Healthy Sensation salad dressings
Kraft Free salad dressings
Kraft Taste of Life salad dressing

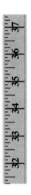

Kraft Vinaigrette salad dressing
Newman's Own Italian Lite salad dressing
Seven Seas Fat-Free Italian salad dressing
Seven Seas Italian with Olive Oil salad dressing
Seven Seas Red Wine Vinegar salad dressing
Seven Seas Viva Italian salad dressing
Weight Watchers salad dressings (all)
Wishbone Fat-Free salad dressings (all)
Wishbone Just Too Good salad dressings (all)

5

Menus for Two Workweeks

Now that you know the basic principles of healthful eating and have lists of food to reference, it's time to plan ahead. In my experience, coping with dietary restrictions when they're written out is much easier than improvising on the fly. The fewer decisions you have to make during the workweek, the less likely you are to cheat on the wrong day.

To help you out, I've formulated sample menus for ten days. They are not written in stone. You can change them all

you like or write your own, so long as you stick to the healthful foods mentioned and avoid sugar, bread, alcohol and saturated fats.

You can have two or three servings of vegetables at every
meal, if you like, and you can have one-half cup of any whole
grain, cooked any way you like, as a course at any meal.

Feel free to substitute my preferred snacks of fruit and nuts
with a serving of anything that doesn't use one of the four no-
no's listed above. The point is to eat a variety of healthful
foods. Also, remember that unless specified, a serving of most
foods is one-quarter of a dinner plate.

Monday—Day 1

Breakfast
Two eggs, any style (cook with PAM spray)
One medium orange or one-half grapefruit
Coffee or tea (artificial sweetener and/or nonfat
    milk allowed)

Lunch
Four ounces of tuna (packed in water) on a whole-
    grain pita or tortilla. Mix with olive oil or fat-free
    mayonnaise, or mustard or lemon with salt and
    pepper.
Tomato and lettuce
A serving of any other vegetable
Diet iced tea or water with fresh lemon and
    sweetener

Snack
One handful of peanuts (fresh, dry-roasted, no salt
    or added oil)

Dinner
Grilled sliced chicken breast strips
Steamed broccoli and peppers
Wild rice

Snack
One cup hot cocoa, sweetened with artificial
    sweetener

Tuesday—Day 2

Breakfast

One container of plain low-fat yogurt (you may use
an artificial sweetener)
One-half cup of blueberries or strawberries
Coffee or tea (artificial sweetener and/or nonfat
milk allowed)

Lunch

Leftover chicken strips from Monday's dinner over
green salad with olive oil and vinegar or fat-free
mayonnaise
One serving of any fruit
Two cookies from the three-star list (see page 71)

Snack

Dr. Paul's Protein Shake (see page 115)

Dinner

Swordfish with Black Olives (see page 92)
Cauliflower with Chive Sauce (see page 113)
One serving of whole-grain couscous

Snack

One cup of strawberries

Wednesday—Day 3

Breakfast

One serving of oatmeal with cinnamon, artificial
    sweetener
Eight ounces of unsweetened orange juice (frozen
    or fresh)
Coffee or tea (artificial sweetener and/or nonfat
    milk allowed)

Lunch

Sliced turkey breast on a tortilla with mustard or
    fat-free mayonnaise, add tomato slices and onion
One serving of any vegetable
Apple

Snack

One low-fat fudge popsicle

Dinner

Two links of turkey or chicken sausage
Pasta (whole-wheat is better) with Quick Tomato
    Sauce (see page 102)
Garden salad with oil and vinegar

Snack

One cup of fresh, unpitted cherries

Thursday—Day 4

Breakfast
Dr. Paul's Protein Shake (see page 115)
Asparagus Pancake (see page 105)

Lunch
Green salad with chicken, salmon or leftover
    swordfish from Tuesday's dinner
Low-fat, no-sugar salad dressing, or oil and vinegar
One serving of low-fat yogurt

Snack
One Oatmeal Custard Bar (see page 103)

Dinner
Pork Loin with Apple and Onions (see page 94)
Yams
Kale or collard greens

Snack
One slice of watermelon

Friday—Day 5

Breakfast

Canadian bacon or turkey bacon
Two eggs, any style (cook with PAM spray)
Coffee or tea (artificial sweetener and/or nonfat
    milk allowed)

Lunch

Tacos, using fish, chicken or turkey (see page 99)
Orange, tangerine or one-half grapefruit
One vegetable of choice
One serving of nonfat, plain yogurt (add artificial
    sweetener for taste)

Snack

One low-fat fudge popsicle

Dinner

Baked Fish with Vegetables (see page 88)
Garden salad with low-fat dressing, or oil and
    vinegar
Wild rice

Snack

One nectarine

Monday—Day 6

Breakfast

Spaghetti Squash Frittata (see page 101)
One-half cup of any berries
Coffee or tea (artificial sweetener and/or nonfat
    milk allowed)

Lunch

Turkey-Rice Salad (see page 97)
One fruit of choice
One-half pint of skim milk

Snack

One handful of peanuts

Dinner

Roasted chicken breast
Broccoli
Sweet potatoes

Snack

One serving of any fruit

Tuesday—Day 7

Breakfast
Two-egg omelet made with a vegetable or low-fat
    cheese
One-half grapefruit
Coffee or tea (artificial sweetener and/or nonfat
    milk allowed)

Lunch
Spanish Omelet (see page 106)
Apple or pear

Snack
Low-carb protein bar

Dinner
Two or three Ground-Turkey Sloppy Joes in Ortega
    taco shells (see page 111) with skim mozzarella
    cheese, salsa, lettuce and olives
One serving of whole grain rice

Snack
One sugar-free, low-fat pudding

Wednesday—Day 8

Breakfast
One-half cup of high-fiber cereal
One-half cup of berries
Coffee or tea (artificial sweetener and/or nonfat
    milk allowed)

Lunch
Chicken salad made from roasted chicken leftovers
    mixed with low-fat mayonnaise, 1 teaspoon of
    vinegar, 1/2 teaspoon of Splenda, chopped celery,
    chopped onions (serves one)
Apple or pear

Snack
One container of plain, low-fat yogurt (use artificial
    sweetener to taste)

Dinner
Baked pork loin chop
Wild rice
Green or yellow bell peppers

Snack
One-half cup of raspberries served in 1/2 cup of low-
    fat milk

READER/CUSTOMER CARE SURVEY

We care about your opinions! Please take a moment to fill out our online Reader Survey at **http://survey.hcibooks.com.**
As a **"THANK YOU"** you will receive a **VALUABLE INSTANT COUPON** towards future book purchases as well as a **SPECIAL GIFT** available only online! Or, you may mail this card back to us and we will send you a copy of our exciting catalog with your valuable coupon inside.

(PLEASE PRINT IN ALL CAPS)

First Name	M.I.	Last Name

Address		City

State	Zip	Email

1. Gender
- ☐ Female ☐ Male

2. Age
- ☐ 8 or younger
- ☐ 9-12 ☐ 13-16
- ☐ 17-20 ☐ 21-30
- ☐ 31+

3. Did you receive this book as a gift?
- ☐ Yes ☐ No

4. Annual Household Income
- ☐ under $25,000
- ☐ $25,000 - $34,999
- ☐ $35,000 - $49,999
- ☐ $50,000 - $74,999
- ☐ over $75,000

5. What are the ages of the children living in your house?
- ☐ 0 - 14 ☐ 15+

6. Marital Status
- ☐ Single
- ☐ Married
- ☐ Divorced
- ☐ Widowed

7. How did you find out about the book?
(please choose one)
- ☐ Recommendation
- ☐ Store Display
- ☐ Online
- ☐ Catalog/Mailing
- ☐ Interview/Review

8. Where do you usually buy books?
(please choose one)
- ☐ Bookstore
- ☐ Online
- ☐ Book Club/Mail Order
- ☐ Price Club (Sam's Club, Costco's, etc.)
- ☐ Retail Store (Target, Wal-Mart, etc.)

9. What subject do you enjoy reading about the most?
(please choose one)
- ☐ Parenting/Family
- ☐ Relationships
- ☐ Recovery/Addictions
- ☐ Health/Nutrition
- ☐ Christianity
- ☐ Spirituality/Inspiration
- ☐ Business Self-help
- ☐ Women's Issues
- ☐ Sports

10. What attracts you most to a book?
(please choose one)
- ☐ Title
- ☐ Cover Design
- ☐ Author
- ☐ Content

TAPE IN MIDDLE; DO NOT STAPLE

BUSINESS REPLY MAIL
FIRST-CLASS MAIL PERMIT NO 45 DEERFIELD BEACH, FL

POSTAGE WILL BE PAID BY ADDRESSEE

Health Communications, Inc.
3201 SW 15th Street
Deerfield Beach FL 33442-9875

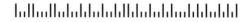

FOLD HERE

Comments

Thursday—Day 9

Breakfast
Scrambled eggs and Swiss cheese
Coffee or tea (artificial sweetener and/or nonfat
  milk allowed)

Lunch
Sliced turkey breast on a tortilla with fat-free
  mayonnaise or mustard
One plum

Snack
Dr. Paul's Protein Shake (see page 115)

Dinner
Salmon with Lime and Lemon Marinade (see page 91)
Green Beans with Pine Nuts (see page 114)

Snack
One low-fat fudge popsicle

Friday—Day 10

Breakfast
Oatmeal
Berries
Nonfat yogurt

Lunch
Tacos using salmon (follow recipe for tacos using
    fish on page 101, substitute leftover salmon from
    dinner last night)

Snack
One Oatmeal Custard Bar (see page 103)

Dinner
Grilled shrimp kebabs with onions, peppers and
    mushrooms
Quinoa

Snack
One peach

6

Weekday Recipes

Baked Fish with Vegetables

One green pepper, sliced
One red pepper, sliced
1 cup radishes, sliced
Two tomatoes, sliced
One green onion, sliced, stopping where the onion turns green
1½ pounds fish fillets—any white fish will do
    (flounder, St. Peter's, catfish, haddock)
¼ teaspoon salt
¼ teaspoon fresh pepper
½ cup fish stock, or chicken stock
¼ teaspoon paprika
1 tablespoon fresh parsley, chopped

Preheat oven to 350 degrees.
Slice all the veggies the same size, so they can cook at the same speed.
Spray the baking dish with nonstick spray.
Place half of the veggies on the bottom of the baking dish.
Season the fish with salt and pepper, and place on top of veggies.
Cover the fish with remaining veggies.
Pour stock, parsley and paprika over dish.
Bake for 20 minutes or until the fish flakes with a fork.

Serves four.

Baked Haddock with Skim Condensed Milk

2 pounds of haddock fillets
One small red onion
One can of diced tomatoes
One can of condensed skim milk
Salt and pepper, to taste
3 tablespoons chopped parsley

Preheat oven to 375 degrees.
Spray the baking dish with nonstick spray.
Place fillets in the bottom of the pan and top with sliced onions.
Top with tomatoes.
Pour condensed skim milk over the fish.
Season with salt, pepper and parsley.
Bake for 15 minutes or until fish flakes with a fork.

Serves six.

Mussels in White Wine

6 pounds of cleaned and de-breaded mussels in the shell
3 cups white wine
3 cups seafood stock
3 tablespoons fresh parsley, chopped

Bring wine to a boil.
Add mussels and reduce heat.
Simmer until mussels open, approximately five minutes.
Serve mussels in a bowl and pour broth over.
Top with fresh, chopped parsley.

Serves six.

Salmon with Lime and Lemon Marinade

2 pounds salmon fillets
¼ cup lemon juice
¼ cup lime juice
1 teaspoon Dijon mustard
3 tablespoons olive oil
Salt and fresh-ground pepper, to taste
1 tablespoon paprika
3 tablespoons parsley, chopped
1 tablespoon garlic-flavored olive oil

Mix together the lemon, lime juice, Dijon mustard and olive oil.
Place cleaned fish in a deep dish, and pour over the lemon and lime
   marinade.
Marinate for 30 minutes, turning once.
Remove from marinade, and add salt and pepper.
Place in a broiler pan that has been sprayed with nonstick spray.
Brush with garlic-flavored olive oil.
Broil for 10 minutes or until fish flakes with a fork.

Serves six.

Swordfish with Black Olives

2 pounds swordfish steaks
One large can of pitted black olives, chopped
3 tablespoons lemon juice
¼ cup fresh parsley, chopped
¼ cup garlic-flavored olive oil
Salt and fresh ground pepper, to taste

Mix the olives, olive oil, salt, pepper, parsley and lemon juice.
Place fish on broiler pan that has been sprayed with nonstick spray.
Brush just the liquid onto the fish, and broil for 10 minutes or until
    fish flakes with a fork.
Spread olive mixture over the cooked fish, and place in the oven with
    the heat turned off, just warming it.

Serves six.

Tuna Steaks with Chopped Tomatoes

Four tuna steaks
Salt and fresh ground pepper, to taste
Lemon juice from one lemon
One small can of seasoned tomatoes, chopped
1 tablespoon olive oil

Season tuna steaks with salt and pepper.
Squeeze on lemon juice.
Heat pan and add olive oil.
Preheat oven to 400 degrees.
Sear tuna on both sides and place pan in oven.
Pour on one can of chopped, seasoned tomatoes.
Bake 7 minutes for rare, 10 minutes for medium-rare, 12 minutes for
    well-done.

Serves four to six.

Pork Loin with Apple and Onions

Four pork loin chops
3 teaspoons Dijon mustard
Salt and fresh ground pepper, to taste
1 tablespoon olive oil
Two small apples, cored, peeled and thinly sliced
Four green onions, chopped
3 tablespoons fresh parsley, chopped
¼ teaspoon poultry seasoning

Preheat broiler.
Using a brush, spread each chop, front and back, with mustard.
Broil until browned on both sides.
While chops are broiling, in a nonstick skillet heat olive oil and add
    apples, onions and seasonings.
Cook until apples are soft, stirring occasionally.
Top cooked pork chop with apples and serve.

Serves four.

Apricot-Glazed Pork Roast

2-pound pork center-loin roast, boneless
Salt and fresh ground pepper, to taste
2 tablespoons olive oil
One minced garlic clove
Two medium peaches or four small apricots blanched, peeled,
    pitted and sliced
½ cup white wine
½ cup apricot spread, made with Splenda
1 tablespoon any hot sauce
1 tablespoon white Lea and Perrins Sauce

Preheat oven to 400 degrees.
Place pork on a rack in a roasting pan.
Using a brush, brush with olive oil.
Sprinkle with salt and pepper, to taste.
Roast for 25 to 30 minutes.
Make the glaze by combining the remaining ingredients in a sauce
    pan and bring to a boil. Reduce heat and simmer until sauce
    thickens.
Top pork with sauce, return to the oven until bubbly and pork is
    glazed, around five minutes.

Serves six.

Lemon-Lime Chicken

Four chicken breasts, boned and skinless
3 tablespoons lemon juice
3 tablespoons lime juice
3 tablespoons fresh chopped parsley
Two cloves garlic, minced
¼ teaspoon onion salt
1 tablespoon fresh minced ginger
½ cup chicken stock
Fresh ground pepper, to taste
Parsley sprigs

Preheat oven to 400 degrees.
Combine lemon, lime juice, seasonings and chicken stock. Add
    chicken and turn to coat. Cover and refrigerate for at least one
    hour, turning chicken at least once.
Bake for 10 minutes, reduce heat to 325 degrees and cook for 15 to
    20 minutes, until chicken is fully cooked.
Garnish with lime slices and parsley.

Serves four.

Turkey-Rice Salad

8 ounces skinned and boned cooked turkey, chilled and diced
1 cup cooked whole-grain rice, chilled
½ cup diced celery
¼ green pepper
¼ red pepper
2 tablespoons green onion, chopped
1 tablespoon low-fat mayonnaise
1 tablespoon fresh parsley, chopped
1 tablespoon plain low-fat yogurt
1 tablespoon lemon juice
½ teaspoon Dijon mustard
Salt and fresh ground pepper, to taste
¼ teaspoon garlic powder
Favorite lettuce

Combine turkey, rice, celery, onion, bell peppers.
Mix well with mayonnaise, parsley, yogurt, lemon juice, mustard, salt,
    pepper and garlic powder.
Cover and refrigerate until chilled.
Toss again before serving.
Serve on lettuce leaves.

Serves four, keeps refrigerated for four days.

Oriental Turkey Salad

Spring-mix greens
6 ounces sliced, cooked turkey breast
4 cups broccoli florets, blanched
One small can of diced tomatoes
3 tablespoons sliced scallions (green onions)
2 teaspoons sesame oil
1 tablespoon olive oil
1 teaspoon soy sauce
1 teaspoon white wine
1 tablespoon minced ginger root

Combine turkey, broccoli, tomato and scallions.
In a container with a tight lid, combine remaining ingredients.
Place lid on tightly and shake well.
Place turkey mixture on top of spring-mix greens.
Drizzle with dressing.

Serves two, keeps refrigerated for four days.

Fish, Chicken or Turkey Tacos

2 teaspoons olive oil
¼ cup red onions, sliced
One clove garlic, minced
1 cup chopped tomatoes
1 cup tomato sauce
Dash of salt, fresh ground pepper, hot sauce and parsley
4 ounces drained tuna, salmon, chicken or turkey
Two taco shells
½ cup lettuce, shredded
2 ounces low-fat cheddar cheese, shredded

Heat oil in skillet.
Add onions and garlic, sauté until onions are soft (about 5 minutes).
Add tomatoes and sauce and seasonings to skillet.
Cook about 5 minutes, stirring occasionally.
Stir in tuna and heat.
Fill each taco shell with one-half the tuna mixture, 1 ounce of cheese
    and ¼ cup of lettuce.

Serves two.

Scrambled Eggs with Smoked Salmon

Two large eggs
1 tablespoon condensed skim milk
Fresh chopped dill or basil, to taste
Salt and fresh ground pepper, to taste
2 tablespoons olive oil
1 ounce nonfat or low-fat cream cheese
$\frac{1}{2}$ to 1 ounce smoked salmon
Six to eight slices cucumber, cut on the diagonal
Lemon or lime juice
Pinch of paprika
Fresh limes or lemons (optional)

Whisk eggs with condensed skim milk.
Add fresh chopped dill, and salt and pepper to taste.
Heat olive oil in a nonstick pan.
Add eggs and scramble over low-medium heat, stirring constantly
    from the outside in. When eggs are halfway set, add cream cheese,
    and stir until almost done.
Add chopped smoked salmon at the end, and turn off heat (eggs
    should still be moist). Serve with cucumber slices, drizzled with
    lemon or lime juice, and a dusting of paprika.

Serves one.

Spaghetti Squash Frittata

1 cup spaghetti squash, cooked
Four eggs, lightly beaten
3 tablespoons Italian parsley, chopped
1 tablespoon grated Parmesan
$\frac{1}{2}$ cup red onion, finely chopped
One garlic clove, minced
$\frac{1}{2}$ teaspoon salt
$\frac{1}{2}$ teaspoon pepper
$\frac{1}{8}$ teaspoon cayenne
1 tablespoon olive oil

Preheat broiler.
Combine all ingredients in a large mixing bowl.
Heat olive oil in a large skillet.
Pour mixture into skillet, cook over low heat for 12 to 15 minutes.
Transfer to broiler for 2 to 3 minutes or until top is browned.

Serves six.

Quick Tomato Sauce

2 teaspoons olive oil
½ cup onions, sliced
Half-clove garlic, chopped
2 cups drained, canned whole tomatoes (smash with your fingers)
½ teaspoon fresh oregano leaves
½ teaspoon fresh basil
½ teaspoon Splenda

Heat olive oil.
Add onions and garlic, sauté until onions are just tender (about 4
    minutes). Set aside.
In a small saucepan, combine tomatoes and seasonings, cook over
    medium heat 10 minutes. Add onion mixture and cook 5 minutes
    more.
Serve over whole-wheat pasta or your favorite freshly cooked fish,
    chicken or spaghetti squash.

Serves two.

Oatmeal Custard Bars

2¾ cups water
1 cup uncooked rolled oats
Two eggs
¼ cup Splenda
1⅓ cups skim milk
¼ teaspoon vanilla extract
⅛ teaspoon salt
⅓ cup dried fruit (your choice)
½ teaspoon cinnamon
Vegetable oil cooking spray

Preheat oven to 350 degrees.

Boil water and stir in oats. Return to a boil, then reduce heat and continue to boil. Cook uncovered for about one minute, stirring occasionally. Remove from heat. Cover and set aside.

In a large bowl, mix the eggs, Splenda, vanilla extract, skim milk and salt.

Add cooked oatmeal, dried fruit and cinnamon to egg mixture and mix well.

Pour mixture into an 8-inch square pan, coated with vegetable oil spray. Place pan in larger pan of hot water.

Bake for one hour or until completely set. Cool and cut into bars to serve.

Serves four.

Scrambled Eggs and Swiss Cheese

1 teaspoon olive oil
Two eggs
One each small red and green pepper, sliced
One scallion, chopped
1 ounce low-fat Swiss cheese
Black pepper and a pinch of salt
Dash of hot sauce

Heat oil in a nonstick skillet.
Add sliced peppers, cook for 2 minutes.
Dice cheese into small pieces, and in a bowl combine with the eggs, scallion, salt, pepper and hot sauce.
Add mixture to skillet and cook, mixing with a fork, for about 2 minutes.

Serves one.

Asparagus Pancake

Four to six stalks asparagus, cooked
Four eggs
Salt and fresh ground pepper, to taste
1 teaspoon hot sauce
1 teaspoon olive oil

Put all ingredients in a blender, blend at high speed until smooth and
    creamy (2 to 3 minutes).
Pour into a heated frying pan with oil in it.
Cook one side until done.
Turn over and cook, or brown top side under broiler.
Serve warm.

Serves two.

Spanish Omelet

One small red onion
Half each small green and red pepper, chopped
Two ribs of celery, chopped
Four eggs, separated
1 teaspoon salt
One small can drained, diced tomatoes
½ cup dried skim milk
1 tablespoon olive oil
1 tablespoon fresh ground pepper
1 tablespoon parsley, chopped
1 tablespoon dried oregano

Combine onion, red and green peppers, and celery.
Cook in small amount of boiling water until tender. Drain off any liquid.
Add salt, tomatoes and milk powder to egg yellows. Beat well.
Beat egg whites until stiff but not dry.
Fold egg whites in the beaten egg-yellow mixture and add the cooked
    veggies last.
Heat pan with olive oil.
Pour mixture into heated frying pan. Top with the spices.
Cook over low heat until lightly brown on bottom (about 10 minutes).
Bake in a 350-degree oven until top is brown (10–15 minutes).
Crease omelet through the middle, fold over and roll onto a hot platter.

Serves six.

Sautéed Cabbage and Spinach

Half a medium-size head of green cabbage
Half a medium-size head of purple cabbage
1 teaspoon salt
½ teaspoon Splenda
One 10-ounce bag of spinach
1 tablespoon olive oil

Core and coarsely slice cabbages. In a 5-quart Dutch oven over high
heat, add olive oil to heated pan, cook cabbage, salt and Splenda
until cabbage is tender-crisp, stirring frequently.
Add spinach and cook an additional minute, stirring constantly.

Serves four.

Broiled Eggplant

One garlic clove, minced
Two scallions, chopped
$\frac{1}{2}$ teaspoon salt
Fresh ground pepper, to taste
$\frac{1}{4}$ cup olive oil
One medium eggplant

Mix garlic, scallions, salt, pepper and oil.
Peel eggplant and cut into $\frac{1}{2}$ -inch slices.
Place eggplant on a baking sheet that has been treated with a non-stick spray.
Brush surface of eggplant with olive oil mixture.
Broil about 5 inches from heat, for at least 5 minutes.
Turn slices over, brush with oil mixture.
Broil until tender, about 2 minutes longer.
Serve plain or with tomato sauce.

Serves two to four.

Braised Endive

Eight heads of endive
Juice from one-half lemon
4 tablespoons garlic-flavored olive oil
1 teaspoon salt
Fresh ground pepper, to taste
½ cup chicken stock
1 teaspoon Splenda
1 tablespoon olive oil

Trim off endive and discard any discolored leaves.
Place leaves in one layer in a heavy skillet.
Add lemon juice, olive oil, chicken stock and Splenda to skillet.
Cover and bring to a boil. Cook over moderate heat for 25 to 30 minutes, until endive is tender.
Drain and remove any excess moisture.
Heat 1 tablespoon olive oil in skillet and brown the endive on all sides. They should turn a light caramel color when cooked.

Serves four.

Turkey-Stuffed Green Peppers

1½ pounds ground turkey
One egg, beaten
Four to six medium peppers—red, green or yellow
Salt and fresh ground pepper, to taste
3 tablespoons fresh parsley, chopped
1 teaspoon onion powder
1 teaspoon cumin
1 teaspoon garlic powder
3 cups tomato sauce

Cut tops off peppers, clean out seeds and parboil until softened. Drain on towels.
Preheat oven to 400 degrees.
While peppers are boiling, mix all ingredients together well.
Stuff peppers using an ice-cream scoop.
Pour half the tomato sauce in bottom of a baking pan that has been treated with nonstick spray.
Place peppers on pan, top with remaining tomato sauce.
Bake for 45 minutes or until meat is completely cooked.

Serves four to six.

Ground-Turkey Sloppy Joes

1½ pounds ground turkey
One medium red onion, chopped
One small green pepper, chopped
One small red pepper, chopped
¼ cup sweet pickle relish, sweetened with Splenda
¾ cup ketchup, sweetened with Splenda
1 tablespoon chili powder
1 teaspoon garlic powder
1 teaspoon cumin
1 teaspoon paprika
¼ cup chicken broth
1 tablespoon olive oil

In a large skillet over medium-high, heat olive oil.
Add onions and peppers, and cook for 5 minutes.
Add turkey and cook until turkey is no longer pink.
Drain off any liquid.
Add remaining ingredients and bring to a boil.
Reduce heat to low and simmer for 30 minutes.

Serves six to eight.

Plum Ratatouille

1 tablespoon olive oil
One large eggplant, diced
Three medium zucchini, sliced
One medium red onion, chopped
One 28-ounce can of diced tomatoes
Four fresh plums, cut into wedges, about 2 cups
One clove garlic, minced
2 teaspoons dried basil leaves, crushed
1½ teaspoons dried oregano leaves, crushed
Salt and fresh ground pepper, to taste
Juice of one lemon

Heat oil over medium heat.
Add eggplant, zucchini and onions, and cook for 15 minutes or until
    tender, stirring occasionally.
Add remaining ingredients except lemon juice, reducing heat to low.
    Cover and cook for about 5 minutes or until plums are tender, stir-
    ring occasionally.
Serve and squeeze lemon juice over top.

Serves four to six.

Cauliflower with Chive Sauce

One head cauliflower, washed with florets cut off at stem
1½ cups plain, nonfat or low-fat yogurt
2 tablespoons chopped fresh chives or one scallion, chopped
1 teaspoon dry mustard

Steam cauliflower over boiling water 7 to 10 minutes or until softened
    and tender.
Combine remaining ingredients in a small bowl.
Microwave sauce for three minutes. Drain cauliflower and pour sauce
    over top.

Serves six.

Green Beans with Pine Nuts

1 pound fresh green beans, with stem ends removed
2 tablespoons olive oil
½ teaspoon garlic salt
1 teaspoon oregano
Fresh ground pepper, to taste
3 tablespoons pine nuts

Cook green beans in unsalted water for 7 minutes or until crisp-
    tender. Drain and run cold water over top to stop cooking.
Heat 1 tablespoon of oil in pan over medium heat.
Add pine nuts to pan and cook until golden brown.
Add remaining ingredients to pan and pour over cooked green beans,
    tossing until completely coated.

Serves four.

Dr. Paul's Protein Shake

One single-serving package of Whey Tech or EAS protein powder
    (available at health-food stores)
Two ice-cream scoops of plain, nonfat yogurt
$\frac{1}{2}$ to 1 cup fresh berries
$\frac{1}{2}$ teaspoon Splenda
Four ice cubes

Blend everything together in a blender. You can adjust the amount of
    Splenda and berries to please your own palate.

Serves one.

7

Cheating for
Special Occasions:
The Four-F Plan for
Fast Weight Loss

W here weight loss is concerned, special events and occasions fall into two broad categories: those for which you need to lose weight in an impossibly short amount of time, such as weddings, high-school reunions and days at the beach; and those that seem specially designed to make you gain weight, such as holiday celebrations, dinner parties and nights out on the town.

Sometimes, of course, there's crossover. For that Caribbean cruise next month, for example, you'll need to slim down super-quickly to fit into the form-hugging little bandeau you bought on sale from the A. B. Lambdin catalog at the end of last summer. Then, like a reward for looking the best you've ever looked in your life, on your first night at sea you'll be introduced to a buffet that offers enough high-calorie foods drenched in sauces, creams and butter to sink the ship.

As self-help gurus the world over have pointed out since the invention of the printing press, you can't always change what the world brings you, but you can change your own attitudes and actions in response to it. Holidays and celebrations will forever come to tempt you. Vacations will loom. And summer will show up with the inevitability of, well, the seasons. So, what do you do?

For one, if you need to speed up your weight loss to meet an impossible deadline, you can choose between two strategies.

- **You can keep doing what you've been doing.** You don't really have to do anything but follow the Cheater's Diet. You won't speed up your weight loss to meet the Memorial Day swimsuit deadline, but you will continue to lose, and you may find that you're delighted with the way you look when that big day finally arrives.

- **You can take special measures.** This choice is for someone who wants quick, dramatic results for a special occasion. Know beforehand, however, that they will come at a cost. Yes, you can lose ten to fifteen extra pounds in just a few weeks, but for that brief period of time, you won't be allowed to cheat. No chocolate, no wine, no cinnamon buns. Sorry. And you'll need to make a promise to yourself—in fact, a sacred oath: You'll return to the Cheater's Diet once you've reached your goal.

A New Strategy

Extreme outcomes require extreme measures. The routine I'm about to recommend isn't easy. That's why I don't suggest you try it as a long-term diet strategy. Although the eating plan below, what I call the Four-F Plan, may be great for nudging that scale pointer toward the left, it is extremely difficult to stick with for more than a few weeks. Why? It's inconvenient and eventually becomes unbearably boring.

I'm warning you about this now because your results after a few weeks may tempt you to try and stick with the Four-F plan. Don't do it. After a while, you'll begin to feel deprived and decide it's time to reward yourself with a little cheating— maybe a full plate of pasta and bread followed by a hot-fudge sundae. (I'm not kidding; people actually do that.) The problem is, that's *undisciplined* cheating, not cheating on a regular schedule. The first time won't cause much damage, but without even realizing what you're doing, you'll gradually slide down the slippery slope to giving in whenever temptation arises. At that point, you may as well make a trip to the attic and retrieve all those plus-size clothes you thought you'd mothballed forever.

So now, I want you to reaffirm the promise you made to yourself a few moments ago: As soon as you reach your goal, you'll go back to your weekend cheating schedule.

The Four Fs of Fast Weight Loss

The four Fs in the Four-F Plan stand for the four elements that I list for my patients when they want to speed up weight loss in the short term. Although this approach can be inconvenient and boring, it's perfectly healthful. There is no starvation, marathon running or liquid diet involved—just some temporary adjustments to your eating plan. The four Fs are:

1. **Frequent Small Meals.** Eat small amounts of food five or six times per day, which has the effect of keeping insulin levels relatively steady. Other diets recommend eating this way all of the time, but to be honest, trying to fit in time for six meals every day can be a pain in the neck. If you can get yourself to do it for a month or two, however, you'll be pleased with the results.

   Here's a sample eating plan for one day:

   8 A.M. Breakfast of two eggs, any style, cooked with canola or olive oil spray. Coffee or tea.
   10 A.M. A small apple or citrus fruit.
   Noon. Tuna with lemon or fat-free mayonnaise, lettuce and tomato. Unsweetened applesauce.
   2 P.M. Sixteen almonds, peanuts or walnuts.
   4 P.M. One serving of nonfat yogurt.
   6 P.M. Four to six ounces of salmon (broiled or fried in canola oil). Small pear, two vegetables from the regular weekday list on pages 63–64. One serving of dessert from the list on pages 47–50.

   This schedule should help you maintain a feeling of fullness, keep your calorie intake low and stoke your metabolism. In fact, you'll run like a high-octane metabolic machine.

2. **Fluids.** Most of us don't drink enough fluids, and that slows down weight loss. Why? When the kidneys, whose job is removing waste from the bloodstream, don't get

enough water, they don't function properly. Something has to pick up the slack, so that job goes to the liver. Among the liver's normal functions is turning fat into a form that your body can use as fuel. When the liver is distracted by doing the job of the dehydrated kidneys, however, it can't devote as much effort to its own work, fuel manufacturing, so more fat remains unused. Obviously, if you want to increase efficient weight loss, you need healthy, well-hydrated kidneys doing their own work efficiently.

For best results, drink at least two quarts (eight cups) of fluid per day plus an extra cup for every 3.5 points your BMI exceeds 25. At first, you'll run to the bathroom more often than you'd like, but in a few days, things will settle down, and your liver and kidneys will begin doing their job the way they're supposed to.

When I say fluids, I don't mean alcohol. Alcohol dehydrates you, and that's definitely not the effect you want. You're trying to get more fluid into your body, not out of it. Following are some fluids I recommend.

- **Water or flavored waters (sugar-free).** Water is water. You can't beat it.
- **Tea.** Almost all teas are good, but green and black are best. Use sugar substitutes. Simmer bag for about five minutes and squeeze for maximal antioxidant effect.
- **Coffee.** People have been trying to find something bad about coffee for decades, but, instead, researchers keep coming up with positives, and caffeine may actually stimulate faster weight loss. Use

brewed or instant. You can add sugar substitutes and fat-free creamers. Coffee is significantly higher in caffeine than tea and acts as a mild diuretic. Drinking too much of it might dehydrate you, so limit your consumption to one or two cups a day.

- **Lemonade.** Make your own with fresh-squeezed lemon and sweeteners.
- **Diet soda.** Not great, but better than regular soda.
- **Soup.** Very nourishing as well as filling, and also counts as a fluid. Soup can be eaten as a snack or part of a main meal. Two-minute microwavable soups are now available that you can prepare virtually anywhere. I recommend tomato, vegetable, lentil or chicken noodle.

3. **Fish.** For your three main meals every day, eat your protein first, and eat as much as you like. Eating protein makes you feel sated more quickly, so without even realizing it, you'll find yourself reducing the number of calories you consume at meals. Fish, especially tuna, salmon, sardines and herring, is the best source of protein for good health, but chicken and turkey breast are acceptable options, as are pork loin, turkey sausage and turkey bacon. You can also add a green aquatic vegetable to your diet called spirulina, which has been called "the world's most healthful food." It offers twelve times the protein you get from an equal weight of red meat, and it's the only food other than human mothers' milk that contains an essential fatty acid called gamma linoleic acid (GLA). Your body produces GLA on its own, but if your nutrition isn't up to snuff, you can develop a deficiency. Other

good sources of protein are organic whey and quinoa, two grains you can find at your local health-food store. As for red meat, leave it alone for now.

4. **Fiber.** The last on this list is adding fiber to your meals. The best fibers are found in fruits and whole-grain cereals, and I prefer fruit as a source. I recommend at least one additional fruit serving at every meal, and more, if you prefer. The fruits highest in fiber are apples, pears, plums, cherries, strawberries and prunes. Beans are another good source, and they offer quality protein as well. Try chickpeas, kidney or green-bean salad sprinkled with some vinegar and olive oil. If you like, you can also use a fiber supplement. They come in three forms: powder, pills and chewable. Just follow the directions on the package. Fiber will help you feel full, will relieve constipation, and may lower your cholesterol levels and risk of colon cancer.

If, after all is said and done, you just can't follow this regimen because hunger or cravings are driving you crazy, you may want to add a weight-loss supplement to your regular regimen. Chapter 8 discusses weight-loss supplements.

Coping with Canapés

Whether you've just reached your goal via the Four Fs or you're simply following your regular workday/weekend cheating schedule, holidays and parties can offer a challenge. After all, even when you're cheating, you should stop eating before you're ready to explode, and giving in to binge foods can be a real danger when they're calling out from every tray the caterer sports past your nose. During the holiday season especially, staying on-plan can be tough when you sometimes

ENJOY A CUP O' JOE!

People are quick to condemn coffee as bad for your health. After two decades of research, however, all the evidence has suggested that coffee may actually be good for you—at least in moderation. Studies show that it may lower your risk for type-2 diabetes, reduce your risk of developing gallstones, help prevent colon cancer, lower your chances of developing Parkinson's disease, prevent liver damage in people prone to it, improve your cognitive function, increase your endurance and make you more alert. It's not completely without a downside, of course. Caffeine is mildly addictive and can cause a slight increase in heart rate and blood pressure, as well as occasional irregular heartbeats. Side effects like these, though, show up most often in people who drink many cups a day, so limit yourself to one or two, and enjoy!

find yourself attending more back-to-back celebrations than fit neatly into a thirty-six-hour window at the end of the week.

Here are some tips to help you cope. Don't just read the list and say, "Oh, they sound like good ideas!" Instead, actually give them a try.

Arrive late, leave early. Perhaps it's stating the obvious, but the longer you're standing around food that's free for the taking, the more likely you are to eat too much of it. At a buffet-style dinner party, figure that appetizers will be available for the first hour and dessert for the last. So try to show up for only one or two hours in the middle of the evening. For sit-down dinners, this tactic doesn't work, of course. Instead, you'll need to be very strict with portion control. Remember, divide your plate into four areas and try to fill at least two of them with vegetables. If your host or hostess sees your plate is full, he'll be happy, you'll be happy, and all will be right with the world. If it's not the weekend, skip dessert. People come up with all sorts of bizarre excuses to offer their hosts for turning down this part of the meal. There's no need. Just say, "It looks delicious, and I'd love to try it, but I'm trying to lose weight." Trust me, you're likely to get more sympathy than a puppy that's just bumped its nose.

Eat with a drink in your dominant hand. Actually, fill your dominant hand with anything at all, including someone else's hand. The point is to keep those fingers occupied. People tend to eat with their dominant hand, especially when they're picking food from a table. Using the other one for foraging feels odd and uncomfortable, and makes you remain more aware of what you're doing. The stranger it feels, and the more conscious you are of putting food into your mouth, the more likely you are to keep your eating under control.

Get a little nutty with your veggies. It is a rare party that doesn't offer a veggie plate for folks who are trying to watch their weight, blood sugar or cholesterol levels. Make this the center of your foraging area. I know that eating raw carrots, broccoli and cauliflower isn't exactly filling, which is why this particular approach often doesn't work, so here's another strategy: After you've eaten all the veggies you want, follow up with a single handful of nuts of any variety. Wait for twenty minutes before you eat anything else. By then, your satiety response should kick in, and you'll lose your desire for food. This assumes, of course, that nuts are lying around somewhere for the taking. You may want to hedge your bet by bringing some, secreted away, to the party with you. I know, I know—your friends may think you're a little odd if they see you pulling a baggie full of unsalted pecans out of your pocket. So do it when they're not looking.

Socialize. Some people will tell you that, for Americans, eating has become a way of socializing. It's true that we organize social events around food, but we actually tend to interact with others in conversation when we're not eating. The simple fact is that it's hard to talk and eat at the same time. Make that work for you. When you're at a gathering of any kind, make the pleasure of being with friends your first priority. Busy yourself with the joy of getting to know someone. It will take your mind off food.

Lose weight beforehand. One way to handle the continuous feast that goes on from November to January every year is simply to follow the Four Fs in late October and early November until you lose an extra two or three pounds. According to a study in *The New England Journal of Medicine,* the average person gains about one pound over the holiday season. By losing an extra two or three *before* the holidays, you give yourself some wiggle room. So have a good time. Enjoy. *Mangia!* Even if you gain back all the extra weight you lost, you still break even. If you gain back less, you're ahead of the game.

THE RESTAURANT CHALLENGE

Whether you end up at the local fast-food burger joint or a white-linen restaurant that offers nouvelle French cuisine, eating out on a weeknight can severely test your resolve to stick to your weekend-only cheating schedule. To make matters worse, trying to decipher what's healthful on a typical menu can be like trying to look up a phone number blindfolded. Here are some tips to help.

Follow the 50/50 rule. Eat only half of everything on your plate and bag the rest for another time. Half the food means half the calories. You won't be deprived of anything. Restaurants are notorious for offering portions that are way out of proportion to a size that's healthful and satisfying for you.

Order à la carte. You don't want to find yourself looking down at a plate filled with some food that will make you fat and wreck your health. French fries are a good example. They're pure carbohydrate drenched in saturated fat and smothered in salt. And if you get into a test of willpower over them, you'll lose. Ordering each course individually can save you a considerable amount of grief. Go for whole foods and fish or poultry. Pasta should be a small side dish, not a main course. Skip anything that's breaded or battered, and if you need a sauce to liven up your fare, try salsas or relishes.

Look for those cute little hearts. Some restaurants have begun offering menu options that are more healthful for your heart. That means low in fat and, often, sugar, which translates into "good for losing weight."

Stick with soups and salads. Soups are great for satisfying your appetite without loading you up with carbs or fats. Any watery food is. Salads are another great option, although

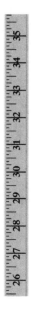

be careful not to load up on croutons or to smother your veggies in creamy dressing. You can quickly turn a salad into a calorie-dense meal if you're not careful.

Order from the appetizer menu. You can make an interesting meal out of appetizers, and because they often comprise small portions, they're a great way to control your food intake. Be careful of the kinds of appetizers you choose, however. A mountain of nachos, cheese and refried beans will not help you stick to your plan.

Tell the server, "No." Say "No" to sugar and bread, and insist that the server check with the chef to make certain what you've ordered doesn't contain butter. Many restaurants, especially expensive ones with great chefs, add gobs of butter to many dishes to enhance the taste.

Eat a small meal before you go out. This is standard advice, and for a good reason—it works. We've all had the experience of shopping on an empty stomach for groceries at the supermarket. You want to buy everything in sight, from popcorn to pickles. (Being hungry in a bakery is even worse, trust me.) If you shop after eating, on the other hand, all those choice goodies that beckon from every shelf leave you cold. You stay true to your shopping list without a second thought. The same principle can act as your guard dog when juicy morsels and tasty tidbits try to sneak up on you at a party. Have a small meal consisting mostly of protein before you leave home. You'll find it helps keep later noshing to a minimum.

Skip the sauces and dips. This is tough advice, I know, but those dips can add significantly to your calorie intake.

If you're going to eat carrots and broccoli spears dipped in blue-cheese sauce, you may as well leave the veggies in peace and attack a pint of chocolate cookie-dough ice cream!

8

Weight-Loss Supplements That Work (and Those That Don't)

When it comes to using medicinal aids for weight loss, whether it's a prescription drug or an over-the-counter supplement from the health store, people seem to divide into three broad groups: those who are ready, willing and able to try anything that will help them move the scale numbers downward; those who are fundamentally against any approach to the problem other than diet and exercise; and those who might be willing to try a diet aid, but are afraid because of all the bad things that they heard have happened in the past with regard to medi-cines and supplements.

My feeling is that being overweight or obese are serious medical problems that can cause severe health consequences, including diseases that lead to disability and death. If you simply can't get weight off no matter how hard you try, or if you sometimes feel too weak to continue following your diet, then I think you need to consider all possibilities, so long as they're safe and effective.

Fear of Fat Burners

In the past, weight-loss medications and supplements either didn't work, or they caused dangerous side effects. Many early hunger suppressants were actually amphetamines, highly addictive drugs that could cause terrible problems if abused, including hallucinations, psychosis, rapid heart beat, elevated blood pressure, heart palpitations, dry mouth, blurry vision, dizziness, tremors, congestive heart failure, seizures and even death.

Then came fen-phen, which seemed to work more effec-tively without the potential for addiction, but eventually some patients who used the combination developed heart valve problems and others a very dangerous condition called pul-monary hypertension. Half of that medicinal duo, fenflu-ramine, turned out to be the culprit, so it is no longer available on the market. Phentermine, the other half, is an effective weight-control medication by itself. It remains available and has proven very safe.

Over-the-counter medications fared no better. One, phenyl-propanolamine (PPA), was sold in pharmacies under the names Dexatrim and Accutrim, among others. It also came with a whole host of side effects, including anxiety, heart palpitations, headache, hallucinations, insomnia, nausea, high blood pressure and other problems that could, in rare cases, even lead to death.

A WEIGHT-LOSS MIRACLE DRUG?

Several studies on a new drug, rimonabant, developed by the French drug-maker Sanofi-Synthelabo, showed that it helps people lose weight and quit smoking! Rimonabant is the first in a new class of drugs, called selective CB1 blockers, that, in addition to lowering weight, specifically reduce abdominal fat, increase HDL cholesterol (good cholesterol), lower triglycerides, significantly improve glucose and insulin levels, and reduce dependence on tobacco. However, don't expect to lose half your current body weight by using this drug or assume you'll never smoke again. People who took rimonabant for a year in a recent study in Europe lost about 10 percent of their body weight and doubled the likelihood that they would successfully quit smoking cigarettes. Those are great results in terms of health benefits, but not miraculous. My expectation is that rimonabant, which will be marketed in the United States under the name Acomplia, will make an important contribution to overall weight-management programs, as I hope the Cheater's Diet will.

Finally, the government recently pulled a dietary supplement, ephedra (also called ma huang or country mallow), off the market because it purportedly caused heart problems and other side effects, including sudden death. I'm not convinced that the government proved its case where this supplement is concerned, but I'm not interested in taking time here to argue the point. The reality is that much of the public perceives ephedra as dangerous, which caused the fear of prescription and over-the-counter medications to spill over and into the arena of natural supplements as well.

I can't blame the public for its fear. I can only say that the long-term results of carrying too much weight are also terrifying and deadly. The answer is not to run from all weight-loss aids, but to determine, first of all, which ones are safe and actually work.

Supplements That Don't Work

Enough weight-loss drugs, over-the-counter medications and supplements are marketed in the United States every year to bury a city, and they all claim to be scientific breakthroughs that work miracles with waistlines. Do they live up to their promises? Let me put it this way: The obesity epidemic in the United States is still growing. If a magic pill existed that could make everyone thin overnight, then we would all be of ideal weight.

The fact is that some products can help, but they don't perform miracles. They can make sticking to your weekday program a little easier, and, if all the plateau-busting strategies I've recommended don't work, sometimes a combination of supplements can help get your body moving again.

On the other hand, many of the weight-loss products you've heard or read about don't work at all, such as these:

Chromium. A few years ago, there was a lot of fanfare around this mineral's supposed ability to reduce fat while building muscle at the same time. The claims were originally made by Gary Evans, a chemist who found a way to synthetically manufacture chromium picolinate, a substance that occurs naturally—in trace amounts—in the human body. Chromium helps move sugar and proteins into the body's cells. Because proteins are the building blocks of muscle, Evans figured that increasing a protein transporter like chromium would naturally increase muscle mass. He had conducted two small studies with college kids. The first group consisted of weight trainers, the second of football players. Evans reported that after giving these guys each 200 micrograms of chromium picolinate a day, they gained, on average, three-and-a-half pounds of muscle while losing a significant amount of body fat. Experts from around the country reviewed the findings and heavily criticized the studies as being seriously flawed. Since then, several other researchers have attempted to duplicate Evans's results, with no success. In short, no credible evidence exists to date that shows chromium can promote weight loss.

Fiber. Eating plenty of fiber in your meals actually will help you to lose weight. Fiber is not absorbed by your system during digestion. Instead, it simply moves from one end of your digestive tract to the other. If nothing else, it helps increase the amount of bulk that you eat, which makes you feel full faster. Taking fiber supplements, however, is not enough. You need to eat whole grains and vegetables. If

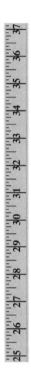

FTC RED FLAGS

Recently, the Federal Trade Commission issued seven guide-lines, which it calls red flags, to help you spot weight-loss scams.

1. Causes weight loss of two pounds or more a week for a month, or more, without dieting or exercise.
2. Causes substantial weight loss, no matter what or how much the consumer eats.
3. Causes permanent weight loss (even when the consumer stops using the product).
4. Blocks the absorption of fat or calories to enable consumers to lose substantial weight.
5. Safely enables consumers to lose more than three pounds per week for more than four weeks.
6. Causes substantial weight loss for all users.
7. Causes substantial weight loss by wearing it on the body or rubbing it into the skin.

you're filling your plate with fare that won't be absorbed, then you're not filling it up with carbohydrates and fats that would be. Therefore, you're automatically lowering calories.

Chitin. One type of fiber in particular, chitin, has been touted in infomercials and exercise magazines as being a particularly powerful aid to weight loss. Chitin is made from the fiber found in the shells of soft-shelled fish, such as shrimp and lobster. The manufacturers claim that chitin will absorb up to twelve times its own weight in fat, including the fat you eat, then carry it harmlessly out of the body. Some evidence does show that chitin can reduce fat absorption by about 8 percent, but it also reduces calcium and protein absorption, and it doesn't seem to have any effect on weight loss. The commercial name of the supplement made from chitin is chitosan. Don't waste your money.

Citrimax. Citrimax is the trade name for an extract of the Malabar Tamarind plant. The chemical name is hydroxyl citric acid (HCA), and the people of Asia have been using it as a food seasoning for centuries. The claim was that this substance causes sugar to be stored in the liver rather than in fat cells, and that it also reduces appetite and lowers cholesterol. Unfortunately, when put to the test, none of the claims proved true. In one study, people taking HCA actually lost less weight than those who took a placebo. In another study—this one done with laboratory animals—males who were given HCA began to show atrophy of the testicles. This product doesn't help you shed pounds and may be dangerous.

Cortisol reducers. Lately, the television airways have been bombarded with infomercials for substances that are supposed to lower your levels of cortisol, a hormone secreted by the adrenal gland in response to stress. Not only do the manufacturers claim that their supplements will help you lose weight by lowering your cortisol levels, but that they will help prevent practically every disease known to man. The logic is that weight loss and other diseases are stress related, so anything that stops or lessens the body's stress response will also help prevent or cure stress-related diseases. It's all nonsense. There is no proof that any over-the-counter medication can affect cortisol levels in any way. A better way to do that would be to take up yoga, meditation or prayer. The Federal Trade Commission agrees with me about this, by the way, and has filed lawsuits against two companies that make these products for making false or unsubstantiated claims.

Herbal remedies. Although a few herbs can help with weight loss, most have no effect. Here is a brief list to avoid, at least so far as losing pounds is concerned:

- St. John's Wort
- Gotu kola
- Kelp
- Garcinia
- Ginkgo
- Parsley
- Dandelion
- Corn silk
- Juniper berries
- Seaweed
- Chickweed
- Fennel
- Ginseng

Orlistat. Also known as Xenecal, research has shown orlistat can help you lose as much as 10 percent of your weight by blocking fat absorption in your body. However, the side effects I've seen in my medical practice proved intolerable to my patients. They included greasy diarrhea, cramping, fecal incontinence and oily discharge. I can't see how anyone could stay on the stuff long enough to lose weight.

Other Debunked "Remedies." The Federal Trade Commission publishes a list of useless weight-loss products. Chromium, Citrimax and diet pills are among them, as well as the following:

- "Lose 30 pounds in 30 days" programs
- Skin patches
- Shoe insoles
- Fat blockers (with the exception of Orlistat)
- Fat magnets, which promise to flush fat out of the body before absorption
- Products containing glucomannan, guar gum, fat emulsifiers or ox-bile extracts
- Bee pollen
- Laxatives
- Electrical muscle stimulators
- Passive-motion exercise devices
- Hunger-suppressing ear cuffs
- Acupuncture devices
- Body wrappings, belts or girdles
- Any of the hundreds of over-the-counter substances the Food and Drug Administration has declared not safe or effective for weight loss

Supplements That Work

In my experience, some supplements do work, but only as part of an overall weight-loss plan. You still have to watch what you eat and be more active. Supplements just make doing so a little easier. By the way, by "work," I mean that a supplement accomplishes the following:

- **Speeds up your metabolism.** Many people with weight problems aren't really overeating; they just don't burn off what they do eat very efficiently. You store too much and metabolize too little. This becomes more of a problem as you get older, or it may be because of a diet you followed too faithfully for too long. Remember, many diets that never allow cheating also cause your metabolism to slow down. So you're eating less, but also burning less. The ideal pill helps you eat less, but burn more.

• **Decreases your appetite, cravings and emotional eating.** You may have a big appetite and feel hungry often, or maybe cravings are your weakness. Others just eat emotionally, from stress or boredom. Whatever the issue, the ideal pill should control it.

• **Increases your energy.** General activity is an important part of weight loss, but many people just don't have the energy to be more active. The ideal pill would boost energy without causing nervousness or insomnia.

So which supplement can do all of this for you? None of them. A combination of ingredients, however, can do the trick. I've listed the top five following this paragraph. All are available at your local health store or on the Internet. You won't get a great result from using any single one of them, but if you take them all regularly, I think you'll be pleased.

Yerba Mate. This is my current favorite. It's an evergreen in the holly family, and its leathery leaves are used as a refreshing tea throughout much of South America. It was used in ancient times by the Indians of Brazil and Paraguay for relief from fatigue. Mate bars are as common in South America as coffee bars are here. Mate is also used as a diuretic and appetite suppressant. In Germany, it's approved for fatigue and is a common weight-loss aid. In France, it's approved for fatigue, weight problems and as a diuretic. It also appears in the British herbal pharmacopoeia as a treatment for headaches, fatigue and weight loss. The active ingredients responsible for its effectiveness are called xanthones, saponins and chlorogenic acid. Although little research is done on nonprescription remedies (because you can't get an exclusive patent on them), so many people had successful experiences with this herb that it became the subject of several studies. In 1999, Swiss researchers performed a study on humans that supported mate's effectiveness in aiding weight loss. They documented an increase in fat burning and an acceleration of metabolism. In the other study, conducted in Denmark, participants lost an average of two pounds a week while taking mate and showed no untoward side effects. In my experience, mate raises fat burning while decreasing hunger and promoting energy.

Dosage: 225 mg twice per day

L-tyrosine. This amino acid is used by the body to make the neurotransmitters dopamine and norepinephrine. It can give energy, help with depression, and greatly ease psychological and physical stress. It is used to make the thyroid hormone thyroxin, which has a significant effect on metabolic rate. When combined with the other ingredients suggested here, it can be an excellent weight-loss aid. It is found naturally in dairy, meats, fish and grains, including wheat germ, ricotta cheese, cottage cheese, pork, chicken, turkey, duck and wild game. You can also take it in a supplement.

Dosage: 250 to 1,000 mg twice per day (increase dosage until you get the desired effect, but do not exceed maximum recommended here).

5 HTP. The most common eating problem among over-weight patients isn't excessive hunger, but food cravings, "emotional" eating and food binges. These are all due to deficiencies of the brain chemical serotonin. As I mentioned before, low levels of this chemical can cause depression, anxiety, PMS and many other disorders. Raising serotonin, along with norepinephrine levels, is essential if you want to control cravings and emotional eating. Among natural supplements, there aren't many products that can raise serotonin levels, but 5 HTP, which comes from the seeds of the griffonia tree in Africa, is certainly the best of them. It has been used to treat depression, fibromyalgia, mood disorders and allergies. Several studies have demonstrated its effectiveness in promoting weight loss. Start with low doses to avoid drowsiness and nausea. Best used in combination with the others listed here.

Dosage: 50 to 100 mg, 20 minutes before each meal

Green Tea Extract. Green tea has been used forever by the Chinese to improve overall well-being and to treat a variety of illnesses, including fatigue, body aches and indigestion. Green tea is rich in antioxidants (EGCG) and bioflavonoids. There is also some evidence that it has antibacterial properties and lowers cholesterol levels. Green tea even blocks the action of certain carcinogens, which lead to cancer. For our purposes, it raises thermogenesis (fat burning) and helps with the metabolism of fat. A recent study in *The American Journal of Clinical Nutrition* found that green tea results in a significant rise in metabolism and fat breakdown. And that's not because of the caffeine. Researchers said that it actually caused a 35 to 43 percent increase in daytime thermogenesis. Just as important, no one had any side effects. Green tea also contains a compound that raises your brain's norepinephrine levels. That, as we've already seen, is a very powerful appetite inhibitor.

Dosage: 200 mg twice per day

Mucuna Pruriens. Dopamine is another very important neurotransmitter. In fact, when you're feeling good, you have the dopamine in your brain to thank because it's the chemical that allows you to feel pleasure. The more you make, the better you feel. If your supplies are low, on the other hand, you feel tired and depressed, and you're more prone to gaining weight. Wouldn't it be great to have a natural product that raises dopamine in the brain? In fact, there's only one pharmaceutical antidepressant that does it—Wellbutrin. Fortunately, however, mucuna pruriens, a natural product very few people know about, contains a significant amount of L-dopa, which converts into dopamine in the body. Dopamine works as an antidepressant, helps stimulate the release of growth hormone, stimulates muscle growth and helps to burn fat. It can also help you feel more energetic.

Dosage: 50 mg twice per day

Needless to say, if you experience any unusual side effects, stop using the supplements immediately. And make sure you let your doctor know about everything you use, whether a prescription drug, over-the-counter medication or herbal remedy. Some herbs, while harmless in themselves, can have untoward reactions if taken along with medications.

9

Aerobic and Anaerobic Cheating

Diet and exercise are always mentioned in the same breath when you talk about weight loss. They're as inseparable as the Bobbsey Twins. But if you like the idea of cheating on your diet and still losing weight, another question has probably begun to tickle the edge of your mind: Can you cheat on exercise, too?

Before answering that, I encourage you to exercise as much as possible. It's great for your health. It helps build muscle, increase strength and stamina, improve heart health, expand lung capacity, develop balance and make joints more flexible. It can also relieve mild to moderate depression, aid digestion and regularity, contribute to preventing certain cancers and greatly improve your appearance.

But if you insist, yes, where weight loss is concerned, you can cheat.

The Real Weight-Loss/ Exercise Connection

The average lean person carries around enough fat to meet his or her energy needs for a couple of months. The average obese person carries around enough fat to meet his or her energy needs for an entire year. To burn that fat, you need to spend more energy than you take in. That's where exercise would seem to come in, right? But hold on a moment. Let's take a closer look at the situation.

Your body has three ways of burning fuel:

- **Basal metabolism.** This is the energy your body uses to maintain and operate all its systems, with the exception of digestion, even when you're quietly lying down and doing nothing else.
- **Food processing.** This is the energy your body uses to digest, absorb and/or expel everything you put into it.
- **Activity.** This is the energy your body uses whenever you do anything that requires the use of voluntary muscles. That means all the moving around that you do in daily life, including exercise.

Basal metabolism and food processing account for about 60 percent of your energy use. Activity accounts for the other 40 percent, of which exercise takes up only a very small fraction. So to be frank, working out doesn't make a huge contribution to weight loss.

DOES EXERCISE ENHANCE WEIGHT LOSS?

A study by the University of Massachusetts showed the difference that exercise can make when you're losing weight. The subjects of the study were divided into four groups. Each group dieted, and three of them did some form of exercise along with their dieting. The group that only dieted lost an average of nine pounds, but 11 percent of that weight was in the form of muscle. The group that both dieted and did aerobic exercise lost an average of ten pounds, and 99 percent of it was fat loss. The group that dieted and did strength training lost an average of nine pounds, and not only was all of the loss from fat, but some muscle was gained in the process. However, the group that dieted and did both aerobic exercise and resistance training lost an average of thirteen pounds, all of it in the form of fat, and gained 4 percent more muscle. The result is clear: A combination of aerobic exercise and resistance training gives the best benefits.

Gym rats are quick to point out that exercising not only uses up energy while you're doing it, but it also raises your metabolic rate. And they're right. If you do vigorous aerobic exercise, such as running or swimming, the activity itself burns calories, and your metabolism automatically speeds up for a few hours afterward. If you do strength-building exercises, such as lifting weights or calisthenics, the new muscle mass you create demands more energy, and your metabolism speeds up to keep that hungry tissue happy.

The problem is that neither type of exercise will make your metabolism speed up enough to make much of a difference where your weight is concerned. If you could jog on a treadmill for a solid, nonstop hour every single day, you might burn enough calories to make a dent in your fat stores, but unfortunately, few people have that kind of time or energy.

So, is exercise totally useless for losing weight? No, though exercise *alone* is not terribly useful for weight loss. When combined with diet, however, exercise is helpful in several ways. First of all, creating more muscle is a good idea for reasons beyond any small increase in basal metabolism that might come about. Muscles have insulin receptors, and more muscle mass means more receptors to use up sugar from the bloodstream. As a result, more sugar gets burned up instead of stored up.

Exercise also encourages the body to burn its fat for energy and discourages it from cannibalizing its own lean tissue. And if done moderately—about thirty minutes a day—it can actually help decrease appetite. Overdoing your workout, on the other hand, can have the opposite effect.

Finally, so long as you keep a strict diet during the week

and cheat only on the weekends, the small energy expenditures you make during your workouts will have a slow but cumulative effect.

NEAT: How Cheating on Exercise Fits into the Picture

Where weight loss, and only weight loss, is concerned, cheating on exercise is easy. To get the beneficial effects of added muscle, you need only work out twice a week. We'll talk about how to do that further on. To burn extra calories on the other five days, however, you can take an entirely different approach. Scientists call it non-exercise activity thermogenesis (NEAT), and it accounts for nearly all of the energy you burn every day beyond basal metabolism and eating expenditures.

How do you do it? You get up and move.

Research has shown that thin people naturally move around about twice as much as overweight people. In fact, that may be exactly how they manage to stay thin. So learn from them. It doesn't matter how you move, just move. Take the dog for a walk. Pace around the room. Move your hands more when you're having a conversation. Walk up the escalator instead of riding it. Rake some leaves. Dust the furniture. Use any excuse to lift yourself out of your comfy chair and to put your limbs in motion. Of if you don't want to get up, fidget. The more you wiggle, the more calories you'll burn. It's that simple.

Critics of low-fat diets like to point out that the current obesity epidemic in the United States started in the 1980s, when low-fat eating reached faddish proportions. But other changes also occurred during that decade, including the popularization of sedentary activities such as computer and video games and the advent of the VCR. Masses of people migrated from agricultural communities and cities to the suburbs, where they tend to drive more and walk less. Manufacturing and other labor-intensive jobs moved overseas, leaving more and more Americans perched at a desk for eight hours a day. In other words, we started spending more time sitting on our rusty-dusties.

TEN NEAT ACTIVITIES

Here are a few ways to boost your daily physical activity as recommended in a U.S. Surgeon General's report. Each activity burns about 150 calories (technically, kilocalories) a day, although the intensity at which you perform them and your weight adjusts that number up or down.

- Washing and waxing a car for 45 to 60 minutes
- Washing windows or floors for 45 to 60 minutes
- Playing volleyball for 45 minutes
- Playing touch football for 30 to 45 minutes
- Gardening for 30 to 45 minutes
- Walking 1¾ miles in 35 minutes (20 min/mile)
- Basketball (shooting baskets) for 30 minutes
- Dancing fast (social) for 30 minutes
- Pushing a stroller 1½ miles in 30 minutes
- Raking leaves for 30 minutes

Since then, the situation has only grown worse. Life is built around convenience. We go to drive-through restaurants and banks. We spend hours in front of television sets and computer monitors. We prefer snowblowers to shovels, and self-propelled lawnmowers to the push kind.

In fact, because of labor-saving devices, scientists estimate that each of us burns, on average, 100 to 200 calories less each day than we did a few decades ago—enough to account for the entire obesity epidemic.

Blame Mother Nature, Not Yourself

"If overweight people don't move around as much as thin people, then aren't they fat simply because they're lazy?" That seems to be an obvious conclusion to draw, but like so many obvious conclusions, it's wrong.

What we now know about NEAT was learned primarily from researchers at the Mayo Clinic, who set up experiments allowing them to measure the amount of energy people spend every day in normal activities. One conclusion these scientists reached was that the amount of NEAT a person performs is due in part to his or her genetic inheritance. The type of job he or she has also exerts a profound effect, as does age and gender. Laziness has little to do with it.

Remember, however, that having a genetic predisposition to being more sedentary does not mean you're sentenced to life as a couch potato. Knowledge is power. What you don't do naturally, you can turn into a habit by conscientious daily repetition. Do anything but sit still, and you won't have to exercise every day to lose weight!

However, because it offers so many other healthful benefits, I still recommend exercising for three hours a week. I absolutely insist that you do it at least two hours per week.

Exercise

People who are out of shape, especially if they are over-weight, become disproportionately overstressed after a small amount of movement. Their muscles are more like old nags than young colts, and, often, chronic dieting has exhausted their systems. To make matters worse, they feel self-conscious and humiliated wearing workout clothes, such as shorts or tights, most of which are clearly designed to compliment lean bodies. All in all, the pain seems much greater than the gain.

That's probably why you've gone off exercise programs in the past. After a month or two of regular workouts, you got up one morning and said to yourself, "I'm too tired. I'm too busy. I'm too . . . whatever." So you skipped that day. Skipping one made skipping another much easier. Pretty soon, your pro-gram disappeared. But as of today, three weekly hours—or at least two—of exercise is one of your long-term goals.

The Right Exercise for You

Low-intensity exercise is a perfectly good way to launch your program, and if you haven't exercised regularly in the last six months, you're not ready for more yet. For now, start with a fifteen-minute slow walk twice a week. As you feel more and more capable, you can gradually build up to forty-five-minute walks (and you would do yourself a world of good if you also increased the number of walks from two to four). It's best to take these walks just after a meal. For some unex-plained reason, the body burns 15 percent more calories if you exercise right after you've eaten. If you exercise just before a meal, on the other hand, you'll dull your appetite a bit, but an hour later you'll rebound and become ravenous.

WEEKLY EXERCISE PLAN

- Work at least one NEAT activity into your day five days per week.

- Go for a walk at least two days per week. If you're not in good physical condition, start with a slow gait for fifteen minutes. Gradually build up to forty-five. You can then increase intensity by walking faster or by traveling over hilly terrain.

- Strength train twenty to thirty minutes, two days per week. Use good form and exercise all major muscle groups, including the back and front of your arms, shoulders, torso (chest, stomach, upper and lower back) and legs. Start with one set of eight to twelve repetitions per exercise. As you become more advanced, increase the number of sets, add a third day and/or change exercises to keep the body guessing.

- Always exercise after you eat, never before. Some research has shown that you may burn up to 15 percent more calories that way.

Should you decide to use weights to increase your strength, I recommend light dumbbells from one to five pounds for starters. Also, find someone who knows what he or she is doing to help you. Join a gym, call a friend, hire a personal trainer or go to the local YMCA or community center. Moving with correct form when working with dumbbells is extremely important, both for good results and for safety.

The same goes for stretching, which is the third and final piece of the puzzle for any good physical fitness program. Stretching is important for helping you stay limber and maintaining a full range of motion in all your extremities. It also helps with balance.

For older adults, Senior Services of Seattle offers an excellent program called *EnhanceFitness* that is becoming available at more and more senior centers around the nation. The program's classes comprise a full range of exercises, including aerobics, strength training and stretching, and they can adjust individual workouts to accommodate even the near-frail.

Myth Busting

As you continue to lose weight on the Cheater's Diet and become more fit, you may decide to move up to more strenuous exercising. This is a good thing, but not necessarily for weight loss.

Aerobic activities such as jogging or playing tennis won't permanently increase your metabolism. If your metabolic rate is slow, it will speed up only during the time you're exercising and for a few hours afterward. If you want to burn a few extra calories, aerobic exercise is great, but don't expect it to deliver more than it can. Use NEAT for that.

Resistance exercise, such as weightlifting, increases your metabolic rate a little. Weightlifting builds muscle. Muscle demands fuel and burns it quickly. Therefore, your metabolic rate goes up, but not enough to make a big difference in your weight loss. However, the more muscle mass you have, the more sugar it will use for fuel—sugar that would have otherwise been stored as fat. This can be very useful in *maintaining* weight loss, but isn't much help in losing the weight in the first place.

Finally, exercise doesn't have to be intense, whether it's aerobic or anaerobic. Just as you can choose to walk for fitness rather than run, you don't have to lift fifty-pound dumbbells to enjoy the benefits of strength training, as I learned a few years ago from my eighty-five-year-old patients at a nursing home in Maryland. Aging causes muscles to waste away. Elderly people can find themselves unable to do simple tasks, such as sitting up on their own or walking across a room. The only therapy that works for people in this condition is muscle building, so I took a group of ten people from the nursing home, with an average age of eighty-five, and conducted a weight-lifting class twice a week with them. We used dumbbells ranging from three to five pounds. Within a few months, all ten people were feeling stronger and enjoyed an improved sense of well-being. One woman gave up her cane as her upper body strength increased. Another was able, for the first time in years, to make her way from her bed to a chair without the aid of a nurse. Very low-intensity exercise obviously had good effects, but just as important, it had no bad effects. Two of my elderly patients had moderate to severe heart disease, but they were able to exercise with no signs of discomfort.

If you're young, you may argue that none of this has anything to do with you. If you're like most overweight people, however, you've been on many diets, most of which severely restricted the amount of food you could eat. You lost weight, but if you weren't exercising, much of that weight loss was due to your body cannibalizing your own muscle tissue. Being young doesn't protect you from that, and you may be weaker and have less stamina than you think. So younger or older, start slow and increase your walking time or lifting weight gradually.

Exercise Tips

The most important tip is to see your health-care provider and get a complete checkup before starting any exercise program. Physical exercise stresses your body, and you need to be sure you have no underlying condition that might make vigorous activity dangerous. After receiving a clean bill of health to begin your exercise regimen, remember that no matter which kind of exercises you do, there are some general rules of thumb for ensuring a safe, healthful and productive experience.

Warm Up and Cool Down

Before starting your routine, walk, jog slowly or perform any other full-body movement that produces a light sweat within eight to ten minutes. Among other benefits, warming your body in this way raises your basal metabolic rate, increases the blood supply to your muscles, makes your muscles more limber, produces lubricating fluid in your joints and gets your heart ready for more intense work. By the way, save your stretching for later. In fact, make it part of your cool-down at the end of your workout. It does not warm up the body, and if you stretch while you're still cold, you can injure yourself.

Cooling down begins with the same type of movements that are good for warming up. Again, they should be light and not too brisk—simply walking is probably the easiest and most practical way to do this. You want to give your pulse and breathing a chance to return gradually to their normal rates so you don't develop any irregularities in your heartbeat. The idea is to let your pulse slowly reduce to 120 or less. Then you can stretch.

Stretch Properly

Not only does stretching make your joints more flexible by teaching the muscles around them to relax, but recent research has shown that it actually increases strength and endurance and improves posture. Most of the stretching you'll do will probably be static, which means you'll get into a stretched position and hold it a while. Here are some points to keep in mind:

- Stretch only until you feel resistance in your muscle, not until you feel pain.
- Don't bounce back and forth, or up and down to get farther into a stretch. Every movement should be slow and controlled.
- Hold each stretch for thirty to sixty seconds. That gives the muscles time to relax and learn to feel comfortable in the stretched position.
- Be patient. Some people become flexible quickly; others take a very long time. There is no rush, and pushing your

body too hard too soon can cause injury.

- Remember to get warm, warm, warm! Don't stretch cold muscles. They can tear. As I mentioned above, this part of your exercise routine is best left until the second half of your cool-down.

Weights

Weightlifting increases muscle mass, improves balance, helps you look great and, of course, increases strength. As a beginner, use dumbbells, not barbells. Weight machines are also good for beginners.

To achieve results, you need to exercise every muscle group in your body twice a week, and never exercise the same muscles on two consecutive days (with the exception of the stomach and calves, which you can exercise as often as you like). Every time you lift a weight, it's called a repetition. A set is a group of repetitions. So if you do one set of twelve repetitions, it means you lift the weight in a particular movement twelve times, and then rest or move on to another exercise. If you're doing a full-body workout, which shouldn't take more than twenty to thirty minutes, do one set (eight to twelve repetitions per set) each for the following muscles:

- Chest
- Upper back
- Lower back
- Shoulders
- Biceps (the tops of your upper arms)
- Triceps (the bottoms of your upper arms)
- Quadriceps (the front of your thighs)

- Hamstrings (the rear of your thighs)
- Buttocks
- Stomach

Lift enough weight to the point that the last two or three repetitions are hard work, not until your muscles fail and you can't complete the last repetition. You're more likely to be sore if you do that, which may discourage you from continuing the routine.

Abdominal exercises are great for strengthening tummy muscles, and doing so helps your balance and provides better back support. But the only thing that will give you a washboard tummy is losing the fat around your middle. High repetitions of classic crunches will do the trick, but do them properly. A knowledgeable friend or trainer can show you the proper technique.

CIRCUIT TRAINING

For a complete workout, do aerobic movements that exercise your heart and increase your stamina (walking, running, swimming, etc.); anaerobic movements that increase your strength and improve your balance (lifting weights, calisthenics, etc.); and stretching movements that increase your flexibility (yoga, etc.). Sound like too much time out of your week? One way to shorten your workout but still achieve maximum benefit is to combine aerobics with strength building. It's called circuit training.

A circuit trainer works out with light weights (a pair of dumbbells with a combined weight of about 10 percent of his or her body weight) with little or no rest period between exercises. I recommend briskly working the following areas of your body for

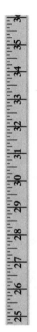

thirty seconds each, either going immediately from one movement to the next or jogging in place for a few seconds in between.

- Chest exercise
- Quadriceps (front of thigh) exercise
- Upper-back exercise
- Hamstring (back of thigh) exercise
- Shoulder exercise
- Calves exercise
- Biceps (front of upper arm) exercise
- Buttocks exercise
- Triceps (back of upper arm) exercise
- Stomach exercise

Within a few weeks, your muscles will be firmer, your waist trimmer, and your stamina will have increased dramatically.

Aerobic Exercise

Aerobic exercises help achieve a number of positive health characteristics. They improve your heart's strength; increase the amount of oxygen your blood can carry by increasing the number of red blood cells; help your heart beat slower, even when you're exercising or doing other strenuous activities; cause new blood vessels to form; lower blood pressure; help lower cholesterol and other fatty substances in the blood; and help your body produce more fat-burning enzymes.

To get the most out of aerobic exercises, they must be a part of your exercise routine more than twice a week. If you pump up your NEAT activities by doing them extra vigorously—take stairs two at a time or climb them as swiftly as you can, for example—you'll get an aerobic effect, which is getting your heart to beat faster and your oxygen intake increased for a few minutes.

If you're raking leaves or cutting the grass, increase your normal speed by a quarter. Even better, walk more whenever you can. Park your car farther from your destination and make up the difference on foot. When you go to the mall, do a quick walk from one end to the other before going into a store. At the supermarket, walk all the way around the inside perimeter once before you start to shop. Boosting your aerobic NEAT time to twenty-five or thirty minutes per day is easy, and it's just as beneficial as mounting a treadmill, stair stepper or any number of aerobic-exercise machines.

Finally, when it comes to exercise of any type, it is important to set goals, whether they be time goals, performance goals or health-improvement goals (physical results). Each time you reach a goal, you'll receive a boost toward continuing your healthful ways.

10

Eclipsing Your Plateau

A weight-loss plateau is a terrible thing to behold. Like a sailing schooner when the wind dies down, one moment you're racing toward your destination, and the next, you're stopped dead in the water. As days, weeks or even months go by without so much as a twitch of the scale pointer, a dieter on a plateau can find herself descending from frustration through depression to despair.

A plateau can be humbling. It is the body revealing its power to have its own way, and it may appear that another

pound can't be lost. But a smart captain never sets sail without a few tricks up her sleeve. Armed with a little knowledge
and ingenuity, she can fire up the back-up engine and cut into
the wind again, or she can avoid the calms altogether.

Cheaters Usually Win

The usual suspect behind a weight-loss plateau is the fact
that when you diet continuously, your body eventually wises
up, makes adjustments and adapts. It becomes extraordinarily
efficient in the way it burns fuel, so it no longer has to siphon
off reserves the way it did when you first shocked it by changing your eating habits.

Most people who founder on a plateau instinctively try to
break free by eating less. Big mistake. First of all, you're
going to get hungry—very hungry. Unless you have no access
to food, starving yourself this way for very long will be
extremely difficult. To make matters worse, your metabolism
tries to become even *more* efficient at spending calories, and
to some extent it will succeed. You may manage to nudge off
another pound or two, but when you finally surrender to your
appetite and start to eat more, your body will be so convinced
it's been ravaged by famine that it will deposit nearly every
extra morsel into the savings account around your waist. The
weight will start to pile back on, and you'll watch, a helpless
onlooker, not knowing what to do.

Some very patient people don't change their eating habits
when the scale refuses to budge. They counsel themselves to
remain patient, and they wait—and wait some more. Sometimes the waiting pays off. The body seems to realize that it's
not in any real jeopardy, so it relaxes a bit and allows some fat

out of the coffers. Many times, however, the waiting doesn't pay off. The scale stops and doesn't budge. The dieter resigns herself to never reaching the weight-loss goal.

Stalled Out

Exactly what you should and need to do when weight-loss stalls out is built right into the Cheater's Diet: Eat more for short periods of time, keeping your metabolism confused and constantly playing catch-up. In fact, there's a strong likelihood that you won't plateau at all, or if you do, that it will last for only a few days. However, if you find yourself sitting high and dry on a plateau, don't despair. While eating too little for too long a time is the most common reason for plateaus, there are other causes.

You're Weighing Too Frequently

You may not be on a plateau at all. You're just paying too much attention to the occasional rise of the scale pointer, which will fluctuate day to day. Just because you're showing more pounds today than yesterday doesn't mean that your fat loss has stalled. Other factors might be responsible. For example, salty food or premenstrual bloating can cause you to retain fluids, which can add several pounds to your weight. Heavy perspiring or voiding, on the other hand, could cause you to drop a few. What you're looking for is a general trend downward instead of day-to-day results. There are a couple of ways to go about this.

One strategy is simply to hold off from weighing yourself more than once a week. That will give you a more realistic picture, so long as you watch the trend for a month or more and don't come to any conclusions from just one or two weigh-ins. The other strategy is to stand on the scale every day and create a line chart on which you track your weight over time. Make the vertical side of your chart represent weight, and the horizontal side, dates. After a few weeks, the end point should be lower than the starting point. Another option is to measure your waist once a week. Because you're losing fat from all over, though, and not just from around your middle, you may not see any significant change for a few weeks. Watching the neck works, too. If your collars are looser or necklaces hang lower, that's a good sign.

You Have Unrealistic Expectations

Ever watched one of these weight-loss "reality" shows that set weekly weight-loss goals for their contestants? "Your goal this week is to lose five pounds." Well, there's nothing "real" about assigning numbers like that. Everyone loses weight at his or her own rate—some a little faster, some a little slower. For good health, no one should lose more than three pounds a week on average. In the beginning, many people lose a large amount of weight in a short time. That's probably the body getting rid of excess water. After that, everything slows down to an average of about 1 percent of an individual's weight per week. That means larger folks will lose a little more, smaller folks a little less. What matters is that, over time, the pounds come off. In fact, some evidence shows that losing weight more slowly may cause your body to cannibalize less muscle and burn more fat, so if you feel like a tortoise racing a bunch of hares, you may be the real winner in the end. In any case, don't confuse slow weight loss with a plateau.

You're Exercising Too Much

Anything that starts using up a lot of stored calories makes the body take notice. If your diet forces you to withdraw too many calories from storage too quickly, as you now know, the body goes into starvation mode, becomes very efficient and starts to replenish its backup systems—your body fat. Exercise can do the same thing. Normally, we expect physical activity to give metabolism a little boost, so you burn body fat at a greater rate than if you were lying down. If you overdo and exercise too much, however, your body feels the calorie drain and tries to plug the leak. You're right back in starvation mode. So if an increase in the amount or intensity of your exercising coincides with a weight-loss plateau, cut back on exercise. For good health, you want to burn about 1,000 calories a week from workouts. That means don't go for more than an hour a day, from the start of your warm-up to the time you hit the shower.

THE BIG PLATEAU

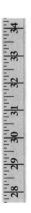

Most plateaus last for a few weeks, at most. For just about everyone, though, the time will come when weeks turn into months, you've tried all the advice, and you still can't lose another pound. Your body is telling you something, so listen to it. You've arrived at your goal. It may not be the goal you originally set for yourself, but that weight was probably unrealistic. Too many people in their forties and fifties think that dieting is the road back to the body of yesterday. Unfortunately, things don't always work out that way. Once your body finds a new set point, almost nothing short of starvation, including medication, will

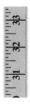

convince it to go lower. The point is to get as much weight off as you can through healthful eating and physical movement. Even a small weight loss can pay big health benefits and make you look a hundred percent better. So give yourself a pat on the back, say, "Well done!" and enjoy the thrill of your victory.

You're a Water Balloon

If you've ever carried a bucket filled with water for any distance, you know how heavy fluid is. It's no lighter when you carry it inside your body tissues, and under the right conditions, those tissues soak it up and hold on to it like a sponge. That's because your body is as smart about water intake as it as about food intake.

If you get thirsty, you store fluid in your cells to keep yourself healthy and hydrated, in the same way you store more calories when you get hungry. So drinking more water can help eliminate retention because greater intake lessens thirst. Often, salty foods (which make you thirsty) make you hold on to water, so put away the salt shaker and stay strictly with whole, fresh, unsalted (all you peanut lovers) foods for a few days.

Also, be sure to exercise. The more you sweat, the better. Finally, eat fruit that contains potassium, a mineral that will make you eliminate water. Cantaloupe, honeydew and bananas meet the criteria, but they're also high in sugar, so save them for the weekends. Instead, eat oranges. If your apparent plateau is actually just water retention, these steps should help. By the way, if you notice unusual swelling from fluid retention in your arms, legs, hands, feet or around your midsection, see your doctor. It can sometimes indicate a serious medical condition.

You're Overstressed

People who plateau are often experiencing high levels of stress. It's usually the bad kind of stress, but it isn't always. Remember, any change in your life can put you in the pressure cooker. Moving to a beautiful new house, getting a promotion, finding the love of your life or winning the lottery can stress you out as much as divorcing your spouse, getting fired or paying your income taxes.

Stress causes several untoward things to happen to your diet. First, many people compulsively eat when they're stressing. They eat even if they're not hungry. Often, they're not even fully aware of what they're doing until they've already packed away more devil's food cake than the devil could on his best day.

Eating this way is probably a result of stress-related drops in brain serotonin levels. Stress also causes the body to release a hormone called cortisol. Cortisol can trigger fat storage and stop weight loss in its tracks. Contrary to claims you see in TV infomercials, however, diet pills that actually turn off cortisol production are figments of some marketer's imagination. The only way to do that is to recognize the high stress in your life and do something about it. If your life seems like a soap opera, work to reconcile conflicts in your personal relationships. If you're having problems with coworkers or bosses, try to open up lines of communication. If you're suffering a loss of some kind, allow yourself to grieve. Exercise, if you're not already doing so. Take some time to meditate, or if you prefer, to pray. And if you find you can't deal with stress on your own, seek professional help.

You're Cheating

You're not waiting for the weekends. The weekdays are hard, I know. Not only do you have work or school, but now you have to diet. So maybe you're picking at leftovers a little more than you should as you clean them from the table. Perhaps you're on autopilot and just pop food into your mouth, chew and swallow before you realize what you're doing. Or maybe you're giving into cravings a bit too often. The problem is that all those little cheats can add up to a big plateau, so you need to find strategies that will help you avoid them. Many books tell you to write down in a food journal everything you consume. That's a good idea, and it works when people actually do it, but they rarely do it. Too much trouble. Here are my suggestions for reducing serious cheating:

- **Take a time-out.** Wait fifteen minutes before succumbing to cravings or food thoughts. Usually, they'll resolve in that time. It takes about the same amount of time to feel sated after you eat, so don't go for second helpings until you've given it that long.
- **Brush after eating.** Giving your teeth a good scour after meals not only keeps them clean, but also discourages you from eating more. Once your mouth feels refreshed, who wants to mix that slightly sweet aftertaste of toothpaste with leftovers from dinner?
- **Get naked.** That's right. Take off all your clothes, sit in front of the mirror and start to eat. I guarantee you that you'll find yourself eating a lot less. After you've done this a couple of times, you may be surprised at how your eating habits begin to change.

You Need More Fat on Your Plate

Dieters often become chronically malnourished because they don't eat enough healthful food, especially fats. Remember, consuming small amounts of fat is absolutely necessary for your body to function normally. When the body doesn't get what it needs, it compensates. If you don't feed it enough fat, it will hold onto the fat it has. You plateau.

The solution is simple: Eat more good fats—at least one extra serving per day. Eat more tuna, eggs, salmon and sardines. Snack on unsalted peanuts more often and all nuts on the weekends. Cook with canola and olive oil. Use Enova oil on vegetables and olive oil on salads. Take fish-oil supplements. This will rev up your metabolism and start your fat burning again. Please, don't be afraid to eat more. So many people on other diets develop a fear of food. It's very sad. So shed a tear for them, then raise your good fats and lose!

You Need More Protein

Eating protein causes weight loss. But let me emphasize that protein doesn't have to be and *shouldn't* be eaten instead of healthful fruits and vegetables. You must eat proteins *at least* three times a day, but if you've reached a plateau, try eating a couple more daily servings. Eating salmon, tuna and soy nuts will raise your good fats and proteins all at once. You might also try protein shakes such as Whey Tech, Myoplex or EAS. Another good choice is low-fat or nonfat yogurt, but make sure it doesn't have any sugar in it. Best to get unsweetened yogurt, then add fruit and/or a sugar substitute to it.

You're Drinking the Wrong Fluids

Some dieters are hyper-aware of what they eat, but don't give much thought to what they drink. Ignoring the effects of beverage consumption on weight loss can be brutal. Sugary juices, colas and specialty coffees can add an enormous calorie count to your day. Alcohol can be a significant weight-loss killer, so save it for the weekends. Both coffee and tea, in moderation, can be extremely healthful, but ditch the sugar and sweeten them with sugar substitutes such as stevia, Splenda, Equal or Sweet 'N Low. If you like fruit juice, squeeze it fresh and don't add sugar. Diet colas are okay in moderation. If you're simply thirsty but want a little taste in your water, add lemon and a sugar substitute.

You're Not Sleeping Enough

If you want to lose weight, you have to be active, but you must also rest. And by "rest," I mean sleep. If you discover that you've been sleeping less, you may have found the cause of your plateau. Researchers who followed 500 people for thirteen years found that those who slept least were the most likely to be obese, because:

- Sleeping less gives you more time to eat.
- Leptin levels in your brain drop when you sleep less. Leptin is a hormone that tells the body to stop storing fat. When your levels are low, your belly, butt and thighs start to grow.
- Loss of sleep is seen by your brain as an attack on your body, and cortisol levels go up as a defense. More cortisol equals less weight loss.

If you're not getting enough sleep, go to bed earlier. If you're having sleep disturbances, talk to your health-care provider about safe ways to deal with the problem.

You're Taking Medication

Many medications can make you gain weight or prevent weight loss. In fact, not only can medicine cause plateaus, it's also one of the more common triggers for raising the set point. As you know, once your set point goes up, getting it back down again can be really tough. Figuring out if medication is to blame for your plateau can be tricky. Sometimes, three months will go by before they start to affect body weight, so it's easy to overlook them when trying to figure out the cause behind a plateau. Here's a partial list of medications that can cause your weight loss to flatten out or even to move in the opposite direction:

- Most antidepressants, except Wellbutrin
- Most antihistamines
- Blood pressure medications, especially beta-blockers and diuretics
- Migraine prevention medications, like Verapamil, beta-blockers and all anti-convulsants
- The newer GERD drugs, like Protonix, Prevacid and Aciphex
- Anti-psychotics and bipolar medications
- Oral hypoglycemic agents
- Corticosteroids, such as Prednisone

Obviously, medications don't contain calories, but they do trigger the weight-loss process—possibly by "turning on" obesity genes. If no other reason seems to explain your plateau, look to your medicine cabinet and consult your health-care provider.

Listen to Your Body's Wisdom

If you reach a plateau and nothing you do restarts your fat burning, your body may be telling you that you are where need to be. Don't fret over it, and don't be disappointed. I have actually had patients come into my office who set high goals for themselves, say 100 pounds, lose 97, and then nosedive into deep depression or flare into a rage because they couldn't get those last three pounds off. The scale is a tool. Don't let it enslave you.

Instead, celebrate. You've accomplished a huge goal. You've gotten your body to a healthier state, you feel better and your clothes look fantastic on you. It's time to be proud and to show off your new self. So go for it!

11

Questions, Anyone?

This chapter includes some of the most common questions I hear from my patients. You'll find the answers are helpful in that they expand on some of the ideas in this book and touch on a few new ones. By this point, you have a good idea what it takes to succeed with the Cheater's Diet, and as you conclude this discussion, be confident that your future holds a lifetime of great eating, fun cheating and weight-loss success!

Q: **Which starches are safe to eat on weekdays and which ones are okay on weekends?**

A: Whole grains are clearly best, and you can add them to recipes or cook one serving as a separate course at any meal. Breads, however, are too fattening to eat on weekdays. This is especially true of lightweight white breads. Heavy, dense and dark breads are better for you—and generally are far more flavorful—but save those for the weekends. Pasta, yams and whole-grain rice are fine in moderation—one serving per meal.

When Saturday comes, you can indulge yourself in white potatoes, white rice and white bread, but be reasonable—no more than three servings a day. In the case of bread, one serving equals one slice. For the others, use the divided-plate method. Corn, which is high in sugar, is a weekend-only treat. One medium ear equals one serving.

Q: **On the weekends, am I restricted to cheating with only the foods listed in this book?**

A: No. You can cheat with *anything* on the weekends, so long as you control your portions and don't binge. However, as a doctor, my strong preference is that my patients make healthful choices. There really are health benefits to consuming beer, wine, chocolate, nuts and cheese in moderation. As for cinnamon buns, well, as I've said, moderation!

Q: **I've noticed that sometimes my waist seems smaller, but the scale hasn't moved. Is that possible?**

A: Some people lose a considerable amount of weight before seeing any change in their waist size, but losing inches before pounds is not at all uncommon. Many of my patients complain that their clothing sizes shrink, but they aren't losing any pounds. I don't know why this is the case. Perhaps exercise tightens loose muscles, which initially has the effect of making the waist more compact, but not everyone who makes this claim exercises regularly. You can be sure, however, that if you're losing inches, the number on the scale will eventually follow. You may have to wait a week or two, but it'll happen. In the meantime, just consider your shrinking waistline to be a good omen of things to come.

Q: **How can you say that exercise has little weight-loss value while everyone else seems to think that it does?**

A: Physical exercise, by itself, is not a very effective way to lose pounds. Infomercials that advertise exercise machines and fitness programs all carry a disclaimer, usually to the effect of, "This product can help with weight loss when used as part of an overall program that includes proper diet." Who's kidding whom here?

The human body has had many thousands of years to evolve ways of fueling physical activity in a very efficient—and miserly—fashion. If it hadn't made those genetic adjustments, people in strenuous lines of work, such as hunters, gatherers and warriors, would've quickly wasted away to nothing. However, exercise does have a role to play in weight management. If you do it regularly, it can help you maintain whatever weight loss you've achieved, and, for some reason we don't quite understand, it can also help the body decide exactly which fat it's going to use first for fuel. For example, recent evidence shows that people who exercise tend to shrink a very dangerous type of fat that builds up around your internal organs.

Remember, if you're physically active enough, you'll trigger Non-Exercise Activity Thermogenesis (NEAT). Many of my patients who like this approach buy strap-on pedometers (available online or at your local sporting-goods store) and commit to taking 10,000 steps every day. Some of these gismos also display the number of calories you burn as you walk over the course of a week.

Q: **Is it true that if you exercise without dieting, you can actually gain weight?**

A: You can indeed gain weight from exercise, and I'm not talking about muscle weight. While moderate exercise—up to an hour a day of concentrated physical activity—can slightly blunt your appetite, too much exercise can increase it. If you eat more, naturally, you're more likely to gain weight. So if you find yourself getting hungry after a workout, change your routine. Strength training is more likely to cause this effect than is aerobic activity, so if you cut back on lifting weights, you can increase your time walking, running or swimming.

Q: **Can an underactive thyroid (hypothyroidism) make me fat?**

A: Although people often believe that their excess weight is the result of a thyroid condition, that's rarely the case. However, if you *do* have an underactive thyroid gland, you may find it extremely difficult to budge the scale. I don't normally measure thyroid levels among my patients unless they seem unable to lose weight no matter what they try, including medications. When a thyroid problem does show up, I prescribe thyroid hormones, but these powerful drugs will *not* in themselves cause weight loss. They simply allow the patient's body to respond normally to food, so a nutritious diet and exercise program are still necessary. Hormonal supplementation of this type may have another beneficial effect—boosting energy, which helps the patient become more active.

Q: **How do medications cause people to gain weight?**

A: The body is a delicate, complex system of chemical balances, and adding more potent substances to the mix can cause the balances to tilt in various directions. One of those directions is weight gain. If a drug raises insulin levels, lowers serotonin levels or intrudes upon the processes of your energy metabolism, you may soon find yourself buying bigger clothes. Unfortunately, sometimes the effect isn't temporary. If you're genetically predisposed to store fat efficiently, many drugs can directly trigger those genes to do their stuff. Your set point will probably go up along with your weight. If that happens, when you finally stop taking the medication, you will not, as you might expect, automatically lose the added pounds. I've listed the most common culprits in chapter 10, but lately I've seen weight gain with many types of medicine, even antibiotics.

Q: **Should I be taking any vitamin/mineral supplements with my meals?**

A: A diet that is low in carbs, moderate in fats and offers lots of variety provides all the basic nutrition you need, but some supplements seem to have additional beneficial health effects. Here are the top five:

1. **Fish-oil capsules (omega-3).** Fish oil is good for your circulatory system, and research has suggested that it may help prevent sudden death due to heart attack. Shoot for one to four capsules per day, taken with food.

2. **Folic acid.** This substance, one of the B vitamins, is important to pregnant women because it prevents certain birth defects in newborns. There is also very strong evidence that it prevents colorectal cancer, bladder cancer, breast cancer associated with alcohol consumption, and stroke. Most important, folic acid lowers the blood levels of an amino acid called homocysteine, which can increase your risk for a heart attack as much as smoking and high cholesterol can. Natural sources of folic acid include asparagus, broccoli, avocados, brussels sprouts, beans, lentils, oranges, turkey, cabbage and spinach. As a supplement, take 800 mg a day.

3. **Lycopene.** This substance can protect against cancers of the prostate, breast, lung, stomach and cervix, among others. Natural sources include tomatoes, pink grapefruit and watermelon. Get as much as you can from food, and always have it either with a meal or right after eating something that contains a little fat (like pizza sauce and cheese). In supplement form, take 10 mg a day at the same time you take a fish-oil capsule.

4. **B-complex vitamins.** Research has linked high levels of B vitamins in the blood with a marked reduction in risk for heart attack. Some people also feel B vitamins can substantially improve mental functioning, but the evidence is controversial. We do know that this group of vitamins affects many, many systems and processes in

the body, and since you excrete what you don't use, you can't overdose on them. Take 100 to 150 mg a day.

5. **Selenium.** This is one of the best-known antioxidants. Studies show it may help protect the immune system, reduce the risk for some cancers and help maintain a healthy heart. Food sources include wheat, broccoli and eggs, among others. If you're going to use a selenium supplement, I recommend taking it along with a selenium-rich food, as this is a substance that may work better in combination with other chemicals found in those foods. Take 200 mg a day.

Q: **Are my genes or my eating behavior responsible for my weight?**

A: Both. Studies have conclusively shown that you can inherit the tendency to gain weight. If you have the genetic predisposition for it and your diet also is poor, you're almost certain to gain weight. On the other hand, if you don't have those genes, you can eat like crazy and never put on a pound. Everyone knows—and resents—people who can do that. But if heredity creates the odds, your behavior and environment determine the actual outcome. If you have a predisposition to gain weight but eat only enough to fulfill your body's needs, you're likely to remain thin, as your behavior and environment will overcome your genetic tendencies. So whatever your genes, take control: Eat a healthful diet and allow yourself a little leeway on the weekends.

Q: **If my genes predisposed me to gain weight, why wasn't I fat as a child?**

A: Other illnesses that are associated with genetic tendencies—such as high blood pressure, diabetes, heart disease and even cancer—often aren't expressed until adulthood. Why? The genes that control them don't "switch on" until later in life. Obesity genes often remain dormant until some event—emotional stress, surgery, medications, pregnancy, a change in career or marriage status—comes along to trigger them. Unfortunately, once they're switched on, you can't switch them off again. From that time forward you'll always have to consciously keep your eating behaviors under control.

Q: **What is a realistic weight-loss goal?**

A: I must hear this question at least three times a day. The answer is different for each person, and it lies within your body. You'll eventually reach a point where weight loss stops, and nothing you do makes it start again. That means you're probably in one of three situations: You've hit a plateau, your weight loss has slowed down, or your weight loss has stopped for good. Only time will tell which is the real answer.

Plateaus last for only a few weeks, at most. But sometimes, people stop losing weight for many months, then suddenly begin losing again. For others, the rate of loss decreases so drastically that they really don't notice they're losing ounce by ounce rather than pound by pound. If this describes your situation, be patient. It may take you a little longer to reach a more healthful weight, but you will get there. For still others, however, your body may have lost as much as it's willing to lose. If you're not as thin as you want to be, this is the time to assess your achievements and be proud of yourself. Losing any weight at all is difficult and will contribute to better health, so you've done a great thing! Now the challenge is keeping what you've won. Don't allow yourself to fall into the trap of believing that you can extend those weekends to every day of the week. It doesn't work that way. Continue with the Cheater's Diet. It's designed to work for a lifetime.

Q: **Is seasonal depression during the fall and winter related to stronger food cravings?**

A: Without sunlight, serotonin levels in the brain begin to drop. The lower your levels of serotonin, the more likely you are to experience cravings, emotional-eating episodes and binges. You're also more likely to become depressed—doctors call this type of depression seasonal affective disorder (SAD). Antidepressants can help relieve the depression—as can vigorous physical exercise—but usually aren't enough to relieve food cravings. For that, you can try the combination of weight-loss supplements I recommend in chapter 8. If your cravings get completely out of control, you may want to see a weight-loss doctor, who may prescribe an anorectic medication such as phentermine in addition to your antidepressant.

Appendix A: Low-Fat Versus Low-Carb

I've said before that you can lose pounds following either a low-fat or low-carb diet, and that over the course of a full year, they perform about equally well. That's not really surprising because when you look at these two diets closely, both fundamentally work in the same way: They cause you to eat fewer calories.

Eating Low-Fat

Low-fat/high-carbohydrate diets came into fashion during the 1980s. Since then, the fad has died down, but much of the medical establishment continues to recommend this as the preferred approach to weight loss. Like anything else, low-fat eating has its pluses and minuses.

What Does "Low-Fat" Mean?

By definition, a very low-fat diet is one that allows you to get less than 10 percent of your daily calorie intake from fat. Some of these diets, though, like the Pritikin Diet and the Ornish Diet to reverse heart disease, try to reduce fat consumption as much as possible. In practical terms, this means a vegetarian diet that also excludes some plant foods, such as nuts and avocados.

I believe that many of these diets, so long as they allow you to eat a wide variety of foods, can be healthful, although there are some very small studies that hint otherwise. Because fats often come wrapped around high-protein foods, some of these diets can be skimpy on protein and nearly always recommend getting your protein from plant sources. That's tricky because it's hard to find complete proteins in any single vegetable or legume, but if you eat plenty of beans, especially soy beans (which have complete proteins) and products made from them, or nonfat dairy products, you should be okay.

What's Good About Low-Fat?

Reducing the amount of saturated fat in your diet supports good health. Studies have shown that doing so reduces your risk for heart disease, stroke and cancer, among other ailments. Dr. Dean Ornish says he has actually reversed circulatory disease in his patients by putting them on a very low-fat diet, a regimen of moderate exercise and a stress-reduction program.

Eating low-fat meals will also help you lose weight. But consuming less fat, by necessity, means eating more carbohydrates. Is that a bad thing? Not necessarily. Vegetables, by definition, are complex carbohydrates, as are whole grains, and they're important to your diet, both for health and weight loss.

A few years ago, the U.S. Department of Agriculture began a study of various diets to see which ones worked and how they affected nutrition and overall health. They determined that low-fat diets produced the lowest body-mass index

(BMI), which means they burned more body fat and spared more muscle. Those that also required high carbohydrate intake provided the best nutrition. Lowering fat consumption may also help prevent some forms of cancer, such as tumors of the breast and colon.

What's Bad About Low-Fat?

Meals that are very low in fat can leave you feeling hungry, so you may find yourself locked into a lifelong struggle of cravings and yearnings for food. Fat and protein sate your appetite more than carbohydrates because they're absorbed more slowly into the system. If a low-fat diet leaves you feeling constantly famished, you're more likely to go looking for food in all the wrong places.

Critics like to point out that the low-fat/high-carb diet craze, which hit the United States in the 1980s, precisely coincided with the beginnings of the obesity epidemic in this country. Cutting fat didn't make people gain weight, of course, but they started eating lots of processed "low-fat" foods to kill their hunger, and that made them gain weight. Why? When manufacturers took out the fat, they replaced it with sugar, and no one minded, at the time. Candy was just dandy—after all, sugar is a carbohydrate, and carbohydrates didn't make you fat. Breads, bagels and pastas are carbohydrates, too. The problem is that carbohydrates, at least in the form of sugar and white flour, do indeed make people fat.

How Do Low-Fat Diets Work?

Low-fat diets work the way other diets do: They lower calorie consumption. A gram of fat contains nine calories. A gram

of vegetables or whole grains contains four. So if you eliminate most of the fat from your diet and replace it with these
other foods, you've cut a huge number of calories from your
daily fare.

Following this sort of diet consistently over time slows
down your metabolism, of course, and thereby slows down
your weight loss. Want to speed it back up so you can burn off
more fat? Cheat on the weekends!

If you're following a low-fat diet and are staunchly against
taking a break from it every week, then skip the high-fat cheat
foods on the weekends and take extra helpings of the foods
you're eating now.

Eating Low-Carb

The current low-carb/high-protein diet craze actually began
in 1972 with the publication of *The New Diet Revolution* by
Dr. Robert Atkins. In it, he argued that carbohydrates were the
real villains of weight gain and that if you cut most of them
out of your diet, you'd end up thinner and healthier. Recent
research has demonstrated that he was right about weight loss.
Low-carb eating can make people thin. The jury is still out on
the "healthier" part, however.

What Does "Low-Carb" Mean?

By definition, a low-carb/high-protein diet allows you to
get no more than 20 percent of your calorie intake from carbohydrates. These diets tend to be high in fat, as they encourage
you to eat protein, much of which comes from animal products marbled with, well, fat.

What constitutes a forbidden carb changes from diet to diet. For some, it simply means cutting out all sugar and white-flour products. For others, it also means not eating foods that have a high glycemic index, which is a number that represents how much your blood sugar level increases immediately after eating. And for some, it means cutting out all grains and most vegetables. These diets have enjoyed phenomenal popularity, despite opposition from the medical establishment, and the fact is, they do seem to help people lose weight rapidly.

What's Good About Low-Carb?

First of all, you lose weight rapidly in the beginning stages of low-carb diets. Seeing the numbers on that digital scale drop quickly over your first two weeks on a weight-loss program can be very encouraging. Doctors will tell you that most of the lost weight is water, but so what? It's still fewer pounds to lug around every place you go, and although you could put those pounds back on just as quickly by drinking a lot of fluids, for some reason, most people don't. Some evidence also suggests that low-carb diets can lower your LDL (bad) cholesterol and help you keep your blood pressure under control. And nearly all the low-carb gurus say that kicking the carbs helps maintain healthful blood sugar levels, although I'm not certain how much real evidence exists to support this claim.

Some proponents claim that this way of eating is probably the most natural for humans. A life of hunting and gathering on the savannahs of Stone Age Africa, they say, would've filled bellies mostly with meat, along with some roots and berries, and maybe a little fruit now and then. Of course, what we don't know is how long those ancient people lived on average. If hungry lions and infectious diseases generally made life a brief affair, having a healthful diet would have been, well, sort of beside the point. Eating to stay alive for twenty years may be a very different proposition from eating to stay alive for ninety.

What's Bad About Low-Carb?

I encourage my patients to eat a wide variety of foods over the course of an entire week. Low-carb diets limit variety and become boring pretty quickly. I'm also not convinced that the health effects of this kind of eating are completely beneficial. Eating high amounts of protein can cause ketosis, a condition in which the blood is overloaded with acidic substances called ketones. In diabetics, this condition can lead to a more serious one called ketoacidosis—a life-threatening emergency—so despite claims that cutting carbs can control blood sugar, I don't recommend that diabetics go low-carb/high-protein.

At least two studies showed that people on low-carb diets actually raised their bad cholesterol, in contradiction to the studies usually quoted by low-carb proponents. At this point, we don't really know what effects low-carb eating may have on that particular risk factor for heart disease. We do, however, have pretty good evidence that eating this way over a long period encourages the arteries to lose elasticity, that is, to harden, which is detrimental to your heart and health.

How Do Low-Carb Diets Work?

High blood sugar causes your pancreas to release more insulin into the bloodstream, and high levels of insulin mean you're storing more fat. The theory behind low-carb weight loss is that eating less sugar keeps your blood levels lower, lessens the amount of insulin you secrete and causes you to store fewer pounds. Whether this is what actually happens is open to argument. There is, in fact, some very recent evidence that suggests that fat in the bloodstream will cause your insulin level to spike and may be an important factor in the development of diabetes.

What we do know is that lowering carbohydrate consumption and increasing consumption of protein and fats sates hunger. In fact, studies show that this kind of eating causes people to lower their calorie consumption to appropriate levels automatically, without even realizing it. You already know, because we've discussed it thoroughly, that lowering calorie levels over time slows down the metabolism. The problem is to speed it up again for more efficient weight loss, and the solution is obvious: cheat on the weekends!

If you're following a low-carb diet and are fanatically opposed to having some chocolate over the weekends, then skip the carbohydrates when you cheat and have a couple of extra hamburgers instead.

Appendix B: Your Doctor's Role in Weight Management

Being overweight creates self-esteem issues for many people, and it's no wonder. You don't need to see studies to know that if you're noticeably overweight, you daily contend with rejection, prejudice and scorn—but the studies are there. In one, a majority of college students claimed they would rather marry a drug dealer or a thief than an obese person.

Even more important, however, are the health problems caused by obesity. Roland Sturm and Kenneth Wells, two researchers from RAND Worldwide, an internationally renowned nonprofit research organization, recently compared the health and economic effects of expanding waistlines with those of daily smoking, excessive drinking and living in poverty.

The results? Obesity was way ahead of the pack in both areas. (Poverty, which can actually increase your risk for obesity—healthful foods are expensive—was next, followed by smoking, then heavy drinking.) Being too heavy significantly increases your risk for heart attack, stroke, arthritis, asthma, sleep apnea, several kinds of cancers (including tumors of the uterus, colon, rectum, ovary, breast, pancreas and prostate, among others), diabetes and injuries due to falls. Many overweight and obese people find themselves coping with the so-called metabolic syndrome (Syndrome X), a constellation of conditions that includes an apple-shaped body, high levels of harmful blood fats such as LDL cholesterol and triglycerides, low levels of helpful ones such as HDL cholesterol, increased blood sugar levels and high blood pressure. Some evidence suggests that this syndrome not only makes you likely to have a heart attack or stroke, but may also increase your risk for developing Alzheimer's disease or other neurological problems. Because carrying around a lot of weight can cause so many associated (co-morbid) conditions, in my opinion it should be treated as a medical problem. That means your doctor has a role to play in your weight management.

No, you don't have to make an appointment with your family physician just because you've decided to go on a diet. If you have five, ten, even twenty pounds to lose, you can certainly do that safely on your own. However, I recommend that you see your doctor if you fall within any of the following categories:

- You're overweight and unable to lose pounds, no matter which diet or exercise plan you follow.
- You're medically obese (BMI > 30) and have not seen a doctor in the past year, and/or you know you have a medical condition associated with being overweight, especially if you're currently taking medications for that condition.
- You're morbidly obese.

You're Overweight and Unable to Lose

No diet works for everyone. Some people respond to cutting back carbs, others to lowering fats, and still others to reducing portion size. A few don't respond to any diet, and no one is sure why. We could simply add that fact to the file marked, "Every person is different from every other person," but that doesn't help people who find themselves in this situation.

An even larger group comprises those who have lost weight several times by dieting, then gained it back and now find it impossible to budge the scale. Research has confirmed that every time we yo-yo, we take a little longer and lose a little less for our efforts than we did the time before. Having an excuse for not losing weight, however—even a really good excuse—won't exempt you from the health problems that overweight people are likely to develop. So if you find yourself in this situation, it may be time for a visit with your health-care provider.

A physician can give your efforts a boost in many ways. He or she can provide oversight, which may help you be more honest about what you're actually doing to lose weight; check for, monitor and treat co-morbid conditions such as high cholesterol or high blood pressure; and/or give you effective weight-loss medications, should you need them.

Unfortunately, your biggest problem may be finding a physician you can work with. Even in these enlightened times, many doctors still view obesity as a problem of willpower rather than a genetic, biochemical illness. You really don't need that kind of attitude in your life. One more person telling you to "walk away from the table and get some exercise" is not going to be of tremendous value in helping you reach your weight-loss goals.

Your best bet is to find someone who has a great deal of experience in treating overweight and obesity, and frankly, that's more likely to be a bariatrician (a weight-loss specialist) than your family doctor. However, don't sell your family practice person or internist short. Talk to him or her about your weight and see where the conversation goes. If you like what you hear, you'll be far happier staying with someone you know than going to a stranger, and family physicians are very familiar with treating co-morbid conditions such as high blood pressure and high blood sugar. If you don't like what you hear, ask for a referral to a specialist or call the offices of other physicians in your area and ask about their approach to weight loss. There is a lack of doctors who generally understand the physiological issues of obesity, and it is critical to your health and weight-loss success that you find someone who does.

That may mean seeing a specialist. I always think it best if a physician is board-certified in his or her particular field. This guarantees that he or she passed a rigorous exam and completed an internship and residency program at a hospital. Unfortunately, there is no board certification for a specialty in weight management. However, doctors who are members of the American Society of Bariatric Physicians (ASBP) have the kind of experience you're looking for. You can call the ASBP for a referral in your area or go to their Web site at *www.asbp.org*. These doctors are devoted to the treatment of obesity, though their approaches can vary significantly. Call ahead and ask if they use diets, meds, liquid supplements, and so on. Check to see if they're associated with any of the local hospitals. I also prefer university training over community hospitals, so in looking for a physician, you might want to ask where he or she did their residency. There are exceptions, of course, but generally, the standards at university programs are higher.

The issue of medications is a thorny one for many people. We all remember how amphetamine abuse came to be a problem for dieters several decades ago, and after that, how fen-phen caused so many people to experience dangerous side effects. Medicine has come a long way since then. We now have safe, effective drugs—anorectics—to help patients with weight management. Because a loss of as little as 5 to 10 percent of your weight can have significant beneficial health effects in terms of co-morbid conditions such as high blood pressure, diabetes and high cholesterol, anorectic drugs are often as useful as medications that are specifically designed to treat these conditions, and usually have far fewer side effects. If you've found a physician who is qualified and interested in treating obesity as a legitimate medical issue, he or she can help you in your choice to use or not use medications.

You're Obese and Haven't Seen a Doctor in the Past Year

If your BMI is 30 or higher (see chapter 2), or you're 20 percent over your ideal body weight, you're medically obese. That's different from being morbidly obese, which means being 50 to 100 percent, or one hundred pounds, over your ideal body weight. Many people who are medically obese think of themselves as being simply a little overweight, but the judgment is not made in terms of how you look. Rather, you're classified by how likely you are to develop medical conditions associated with carrying too much fat on your body.

If you're medically obese, or even overweight (BMI = 25–30), you may need to be under a doctor's care, and the only way you'll know for sure is to see one and ask for a complete physical. This is especially true if you have any unusual symptoms, including, but by no means limited to, shortness of breath, difficulty breathing, chest pain, numbness in your limbs, pins-and-needles sensations anywhere in your body, headaches, blurry or double vision, extreme hunger, extreme thirst, irritability, fatigue, frequent urination, nausea, dizziness, excessive sweating, heart palpitations or an accelerated heartbeat, or any other ache or pain that seems out of the ordinary. All of these are symptoms of various conditions associated with being overweight, especially insulin resistance (pre-diabetes), full-blown type-2 diabetes (the kind you get from being overweight), high blood pressure, and circulatory ailments that could lead to a heart attack or stroke.

If you already know you have a medical condition and are taking medication for it, keeping in touch with your physician carries added importance. Losing weight, especially with conditions like diabetes and high blood pressure, can change your medical requirements. For example, weight loss can gradually cause your blood pressure to drop—a result we normally think of as being very healthful. However, if you continue taking a high dose of medication for your condition while this is happening, you might cause your pressure to go so low that you become dizzy or even pass out. Likewise with diabetes medications. If weight loss makes your blood sugar level drop, medications to make it drop even further might cause you to develop hypoglycemia, or blood sugar that is too low—a dangerous situation that can quickly turn into a medical emergency.

You're Morbidly Obese

In my opinion, morbid obesity constitutes a medical emergency. If you're one hundred pounds overweight (BMI ≥ 40), you need to be under a doctor's care to monitor your health and help you lower your weight. At the very least, you need to follow a strict diet and exercise plan, and probably use medications as well.

In extreme cases, you may even need bariatric surgery, though I'm not a big fan of these procedures. They are major surgeries with major associated risks. Of the 150,000 people who will undergo bariatric surgical procedures this year, 1,500 will die from complications of the operations, even if performed properly from start to finish—which they often are not. However, if your health is degenerating rapidly, you may have no choice. Ninety-nine chances out of a hundred is far better odds than that of end-stage diabetes or malignant blood pressure.

Bariatric surgery works either by making your stomach smaller so you can't eat as much food, or by constructing a gastric bypass that routes food around parts of your small intestine so you can't absorb as much of it. Often, a combination of both procedures is used. Stomach size is reduced either by tying off part of it with a rubber band or by surgically removing a large part of it. The risks of all these operations are about the same, although gastric bypass has a slightly higher risk for causing nutritional deficiencies.

Choosing the right surgeon is extremely important. Here's what to ask:

- **Is the surgeon a member of the American Society of Bariatric Surgeons (ASBS)?** This is the only professional organization for bariatric surgeons in the United States, and it offers specific guidelines for credentialing doctors and hospitals.
- **Is the surgeon board-certified?** Again, these are major surgical procedures. Any doctor performing them should be certified by the American Board of Surgery, which requires a specific course of training, oral and written exams, and re-testing every ten years.
- **How many years has the surgeon been in the bariatric field?** Experience counts. The length of time the surgeon has been in the field is one predictor of how safe you will be in his or her hands.
- **How many of the procedures has the surgeon performed?** This question is related to the previous one and is the strongest predictor of whether or not you're likely to have complications from your surgery. Make certain, also, that procedures of the type you're about to undergo are performed on a regular basis at that hospital.

Remember, too, that surgery is only your first step toward achieving healthful weight. You'll still have to be careful how much you eat, and you will need to choose from a wide variety of healthful foods.

Older Overweight Individuals

If you're over age seventy, the picture becomes a little muddier. The risks associated with obesity change as we grow older. Recent studies suggest that the BMI cutoff for adults over seventy should be slightly higher than for everyone else. In fact, a low BMI (< 20) increases the risk of death among older adults, possibly because of under-nutrition, osteoporosis and fractures due to falling, all of which are associated with low body fat. The Longitudinal Study of Aging, which looked at 7,000 people, showed that a BMI of 30 to 35 for women and 27 to 30 for men was most healthful for people age seventy and older. Many experts now believe it's inappropriate, if not dangerous, to treat elderly people's obesity unless they have health conditions that might be improved through weight loss.

About the Authors

Paul Rivas, M.D., is a graduate of the University of Maryland Medical School and a board-certified internist who has specialized in the treatment of obesity since 1994. He has successfully treated over 15,000 patients and has been interviewed as an expert on obesity on more than fifty radio and television programs, such as *Good Morning America,* and numerous print publications, including *The Wall Street Journal, Cosmopolitan* and the *Los Angeles Times.* Dr. Rivas has also given numerous seminars on managing the condition to health-care providers in the Baltimore, Maryland, area. He is a member of the American Society of Bariatric Physicians and the American Obesity Association. Dr. Rivas's other published books include *Turn Off the Hunger Switch* and *Turn Off the Hunger Switch Naturally.*

E. A. Tremblay has contributed to over one hundred published books as either co-writer or editor. He has held the position of senior editor at two major publishing houses and is coauthor, with Dr. Rivas, of *Turn Off the Hunger Switch* and *Turn Off the Hunger Switch Naturally.* Mr. Tremblay is also the author of two published novels and a biography of biologist Rachel Carson that is written for young adults. He currently serves as editorial director for a public-relations firm outside of Philadelphia, Pennsylvania, is an acquisitions consultant for a publishing house in Houston, Texas, and runs his own editorial consulting firm.

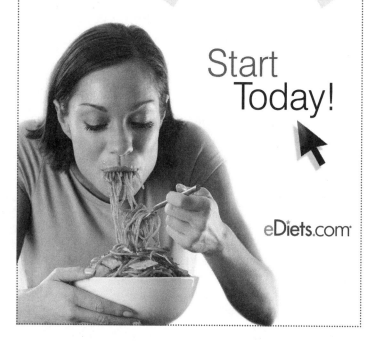